(dis)Honor Thy Mother

(dis)Honor Thy Mother

Daughterhood, Dysfunction and Deliverance

BRIDGETTE PETEET

WILEY

Published by John Wiley & Sons, Inc., Hoboken, New Jersey.

For general information on our other products and services or for technical support, please contact our Customer Care Department within the United States at (800) 762-2974, outside the United States at (317) 572-3993 or fax (317) 572-4002.

Wiley also publishes its books in a variety of electronic formats. Some content that appears in print may not be available in electronic formats. For more information about Wiley products, visit our web site at www.wiley.com.

Library of Congress Cataloging-in-Publication Data Applied for:

Paperback ISBN: 9781394359707
ePDF: 9781394359721
ePUB: 9781394359714

Cover Design: Wiley
Cover Images: © Techzaka/stock.adobe.com, © Mr. Designer/stock.adobe.com, © krecunat/stock.adobe.com, © visualgo/Getty Images

Set in 12/15pt AdobeGaramondPro by Straive, Pondicherry, India
Printed and bound by CPI Group (UK) Ltd, Croydon, CR0 4YY

C9781394359707_261025

To my daughters
May the pinnacle of my life be the valley from which you begin.

Honor thy father and mother; which is the first commandment with promise;
That it may be well with thee, and thou mayest live long on the earth.

Ephesians 6:2–3 (KJV)

Contents

Contents

Main Character List

Bridgette (Bridge, Dr. Peteet): Narrator, principal character; psychologist, professor.

Debra (Mom, Mother): Narrator's mother; former medical assistant, unemployed.

Tony, Sr. (Dad): Narrator's father/Debra's 1st husband; construction business owner.

Damien: Narrator's husband; information technology, chief.

Devon (Dev): Narrator's first youngest sister; operations, manager.

Tanya: Narrator's second youngest sister/biological cousin; entrepreneur, unknown.

Tony, Jr.: Narrator's older brother; construction, unknown.

Granny: Narrator's maternal grandmother/Debra's mother; homemaker, retired.

Pawpaw: Narrator's maternal grandfather/Debra's father; machinist, retired.

Brian: Narrator's maternal uncle; military/government, retired.

April: Narrator's maternal aunt; entrepreneur, unknown.

Tamara: Narrator's stepmother; government, retired.

Owen: Narrator's "foster" brother; unknown.

Dr. V: Narrator's undergraduate professor and mentor.

Dr. Burlew: Narrator's graduate school research mentor.

William: Debra's 2nd husband; automotive assembly.

Ricky: Debra's 3rd husband; formerly incarcerated, unemployed.

Malik: Debra's 4th husband; military, sales.

Cases

"Ashley": A 20-something clinical psychology doctoral graduate student.

"Avery": A 27-year-old Jamaican, separated mother of one; entrepreneur.

"Kaliyah": A 31-year-old African American divorced mother of three; secretary.

"Lynn": A 50-year old White woman, administrative assistant.

"Mia": A 51-year-old single Black female mother of one; firefighter, retired.

"Samantha": A 25-year-old, lesbian woman of unknown "mixed" race, mother of one; teacher.

"Sarah": A 22-year-old Indonesian college student, adopted by White parents.

"Tatiana": A 21-year-old, single, Black/Mexican biracial mother of two; call center agent.

Testimony

"I DON'T EVEN know why you would become a psychologist anyway. I can't see you being any good at that."

Those were the words my mother spoke over me at my farewell party. It was the summer of 2000. I was 22 years old, had just earned my bachelor's degree, and was preparing to move to an unfamiliar city to pursue an M.A./Ph.D. in clinical psychology. Though my mother's traditionally critical words fueled an enduring undercurrent of self-doubt that lingered until my mid-30s, I discovered purpose, direction, and healing through the work that I've done in this field in the two decades since.

I am now a licensed psychologist, twice-tenured university professor, and researcher. Like most psychologists, through providing direct therapy services and supervision, I've counseled hundreds of individuals with a history of childhood maltreatment and abuse. However, along with 23% of other psychologists,[1] I am also a survivor, a broken healer. Within these pages I shed light on the complexities of mother–daughter relationships, the long-term ramifications of maternal maltreatment, and offer healing strategies through personal stories and those of the many courageous women I've counseled over the years.

On the subject of critical and abusive mothers, we meet the discourse with discomfort, skepticism, and minimization, possibly due to the prevailing belief in maternal nurturing and the perception that mothers are inherently selfless caregivers. This reaction is likely a by-product of deeply ingrained gender stereotypes and cultural biases that favor mothers. However, the reality of human experience is far more complex, and it is undeniable that not all mothers conform to these idyllic images. Mothers can display a spectrum of behaviors that inflict harm upon their children, whether physical, emotional, or psychological.[2,3] However, we seldom hold these discussions beyond the confidential confines of therapy. Even in jest, conversations about mothers retain an undertone of seriousness.

During the COVID-19 pandemic quarantine, my close-knit group of girlfriends, Angie, Octaviana, Tiffany, and I, found solace in virtual gatherings, which became a monthly, Friday-afternoon tradition. This particular day, we decided to inject a bit of play into our usual three-hour chats. One friend proposed that we play "One Gotta Go," and the concept was intriguing. Each card presented four options; the challenge was choosing which one had to go. The topics ranged from holiday side dishes like macaroni and cheese, yams, potato salad, and stuffing (the correct answer is potato salad) to deciding which holiday to eliminate. The decisions triggered humorous and heated discussions.

The holiday card asked us to decide between erasing Christmas, Thanksgiving, Your Birthday, or Mother's Day. Without hesitation, I promptly voiced my choice: Mother's Day. Though I am a mother, it seemed like an easy question. No discussion was needed. In my opinion, all the remaining choices were way better. But my nonchalant response was met with silence. This reaction was surprising since, at the time, I was the only mother in the group. Reluctantly, my friends all agreed. Curious about their hesitation, I dug a little deeper.

As a group of clinicians who knew I was drafting this book, my girlfriends were open to further exploring their emotions. A shared sentiment of guilt emerged, a subtle pang of remorse at the idea of even hypothetically slighting their mothers. They were keenly aware of the irrationality of these feelings, yet the discomfort persisted. This experience underscored a powerful truth: the position and reverence accorded to mothers, even within the realm of imagination, wield a profound influence on our emotions and convictions. If we struggled to remove a contrived holiday hypothetically, how could we hope to engage in a candid unraveling of the more complex subject of maternal abuse?

As a brief introduction, adverse childhood experiences or ACEs are a range of abusive events including physical, emotional, and sexual abuse, physical or emotional neglect, and household dysfunction that occurred before the age of 18. More than half (64%) of U.S. adults have had at least one ACE (see Appendix for details).[4] ACEs have been heavily studied and are associated with a host of major negative psychological, behavioral, and health outcomes in adulthood[5]; however, there's been limited focus on those who go on to achieve healthy emotional and personal functioning.

Like me, many of my female clients, and others, have gone on to break the toxic generational cycles of their families. Herein we'll discuss the restorative power of healthy relationships and the benefits of therapy, education, and faith in this infinite recovery process. However, we'll also unpack the silent threats that seem to continuously plague us no matter how much healing work we do—feelings of impostorism.

Many abuse survivors have strived to attain various levels of outward success and internal health, yet beneath the surface, we seem to grapple with the "impostor phenomenon" (IP) or feeling like a fraud despite high levels of achievement. Pauline Rose Clance and Suzanne Imes coined this term in 1978,[6] ironically the year of my birth. In the hundreds of articles that have since been published on the topic, including my own, we understand that these feelings are more prevalent among overachieving women and people of color.[6–8] While IP is not an official psychological syndrome within the guidelines of the *Diagnostic and Statistical Manual of Mental Disorders (DSM)*,[9] it often co-occurs with anxiety and depression.[10] Research also found that IP is associated with perfectionism, neuroticism (anxiety, self-doubt, and emotional instability), and low self-esteem.

Clance and Imes attribute the origins of IP to many factors including internalized societal messages that reinforce the idea that women do not belong in positions of power and leadership.[6] However, I believe that for many women these voices originate a little closer to home. It is said that a mother's words become a child's inner voice. Many daughters have been fortunate enough to have loving and affirming mothers. For these women, their primary battle may be against low societal expectations. However, I and countless other women have endured hypercritical or emotionally abusive and immature mothers. I argue that her words are immensely more powerful.

Anecdotal evidence from social media and my therapy clients suggests that candid conversations about maternal maltreatment rarely transpire. Survivors of maternal abuse, including my clients and me, are not often given space to tell our stories without nearly instantaneous backlash. We are cut off when we attempt to express our feelings. Our mothers ensure their own victimhood and halt conversations with exclamations like, "well, I guess I was the worst mother in the world." Strangers are quick to remind us that "you only get one mother." We are assured that she "did her best" without knowing whether it was true and if it was the case we know it was not enough. Family fast forwards past our pain and push us to forgive. Christianity implores us to "honor thy mother," stopping short of the obligation of parents not to harm their children. It renders our pain invisible.

The external pressure becomes internalized. Brief commentary on our trauma may escape our lips but rapid backpedaling to maternal redemption follows. We self-soothe with statements like, "she stayed" or "she kept a roof over my head" yet it makes the abuse no less true.

Of note, we must use words like "trauma" and "abuse" with care, avoiding casual overuse or dramatization. A friend once said to me, "It's trauma if you believe it's trauma." My immediate response? "Uh, no. Not always." I like to call these my "Bridgette responses"—those unfiltered reactions that slip out before I remember to don my professional hat. Trauma refers to events that fall outside the norm—an accident, a violent crime, neglect, abuse, the death of a loved one, or any other life-altering experience.[11] However, trauma isn't just about the event itself—it's about the potential aftermath, the emotional wreckage that may linger long after. Similarly, abuse and neglect, as part of trauma, involve specific actions or failures to act by caregivers that lead to harm or unmet basic needs in a child. That said, not every difficulty or hurt we encounter is trauma. Some challenges are simply part of being human—a misunderstanding, an offhand comment, or a bad day. While these moments may still leave a mark, they are distinct from the profound wounds of trauma or abuse. Furthermore, few people who experiences a traumatic event go on to develop disorders like posttraumatic stress disorder (PTSD) or other mental health conditions and the majority of people recover naturally with time.[12] Recognizing this distinction allows us to honor the depth of true trauma while framing everyday struggles in an appropriate context. These experiences are often shared only within the confines of therapy.

Clinical psychologists have an ethical mandate to retain the contents of therapy in confidence.[13] In Black (i.e., African American, Caribbean, African) culture in particular, we are socialized not to "air our dirty laundry."[14] Thus, I approached this work with trepidation, violating social and religious norms of respect, secrecy, and silence, and inviting readers into the sanctity of this classified space. Pulling back the curtains of secrecy is delicate work, but one that I believe is beneficial for the greater good. Other women need to know that they are not alone in their experiences. It is time to reclaim our space.

In preparation for this book, I revisited my client session notes. I reviewed my private journals and letters and emails from my mother and dug into the depths of my childhood memories, fully owning that perception and memory are fallible. Rather than a chronological account, I bring the content together thematically to highlight connections and patterns that bleed beyond a strictly sequential timeline.

Psychologists, clinical social workers, counselors, and researchers will benefit from finding new perspectives and resources for clients and populations who have survived abuse. Some names, locations, and identifying characteristics have been changed to protect the privacy of those depicted. I have also obtained consent to share stories when feasible. Dialogue has been reproduced from memory. There will be flaws but I strived for accuracy in everything presented herein.

As we embark on this discussion, you'll encounter stories that may be difficult to hear, moments that might hit close to home, and insights that challenge our preconceived notions. If you become too emotional or distressed as you read, remember that taking a break is okay. In fact, I recommend it. Bookmark the page and, put the book down; press pause. Take a moment to ground yourself by moving to the edge of your chair or standing upright. Press your feet into the floor. Focus on the surface underneath you. Pay attention to the sensations. Notice the pressure or absence of pressure in your toes. Think about your connection to the earth and the stability that it provides. Pause there for as long as you need.[15] Take these breaks as often as necessary, but continue doing the work of understanding or recovery.

Fully reliving your ACEs isn't necessary for optimal wellness, especially without the support of a qualified mental health professional. I encourage survivors to focus on how childhood adversity may affect your present life and relationships, discover new insights, and identify healthier ways to cope. Find the tools within to live past trauma. For those not abused, pause too, but don't stop listening. We need you to hear and accept our experiences as valid.

Breaking the silence around the topic of abusive mothers helps create healthy environments where those affected can find support, validation, and resources to address their experiences. Open conversations challenge societal taboos, encourage empathy, and pave the way for necessary interventions and preventive measures. In the end, through understanding, we may find a glimmer of hope—a chance to break free, heal, and foster healthier relationships, not just with others but with ourselves as well. In healing, we are honorable.

References

1. Feldman-Summers, S., & Pope, K. S. (1994). The experience of "forgetting" childhood abuse: a national survey of psychologists. *Journal of Consulting and Clinical Psychology, 62*(3), 636.

2. Statista. (2025). *Number of child abuse victims in the United States in 2022, by perpetrator relationship.* Child abuse victims by perpetrator relationship U.S. 2022 | Statista

3. U.S. Department of Health & Human Services, Administration for Children and Families, Administration on Children, Youth and Families, Children's Bureau. (2023). *Child maltreatment* 2021. https://www.acf.hhs.gov/cb/data-research/child-maltreatment.

4. Swedo, E. A., Aslam, M. V., Dahlberg, L. L., Niolon, P. H., Guinn, A. S., … Mercy, J. A. (2023). Prevalence of adverse childhood experiences among US adults—behavioral risk factor surveillance system, 2011–2020. *MMWR. Morbidity and Mortality Weekly Report,* 72.

5. Merrick, M. T., Ford, D. C., Ports, K. A., Guinn, A. S., Chen, J., Klevens, J., … Mercy, J. A. (2019). Vital signs: Estimated proportion of adult health problems attributable to adverse childhood experiences and implications for prevention—25 States, 2015–2017. *MMWR. Morbidity and Mortality Weekly Report, 68,* 999–1005. http://dx.doi.org/10.15585/mmwr.mm6844e1

6. Clance, P. R., & Imes, S. A. (1978). The impostor phenomenon in high achieving women: Dynamics and therapeutic interventions. *Psychotherapy: Theory Research and Practice, 15,* 241–247.

7. Ahmed, A., Cruz, T., Kaushal, A., Kobuse, Y., & Wang, K. (2020). Why is there a higher rate of impostor syndrome among BIPOC. *Across the Spectrum of Socioeconomics, 1*(2), 1–17.

8. Cokley, K. O., Bernard, D. L., Stone-Sabali, S., & Awad, G. H. (2023). Impostor phenomenon in racially/ethnically minoritized groups: Current knowledge and future directions. *Annual Review of Clinical Psychology, 19,* 1–26. https://doi.org/10.1146/annurev-clinpsy-071122-030325

9. American Psychiatric Association. (2022). Diagnostic and statistical manual of mental disorders *(DSM 5th ed., text rev.)* https://doi.org/10.1176/appi.books.9780890425787

10. Bravata, D. M., Watts, S. A., Keefer, A. L., Madhusudhan, D. K., Tanya, K. T., Clark, D. M., … Hagg, H. K. (2020). Prevalence, predictors, and treatment of impostor syndrome: A systematic review. *Journal of General Internal Medicine, 35,* 1252–1275.

11. American Psychological Association (APA). (2018). *Trauma. APA Dictionary of Psychology.* https://dictionary.apa.org/trauma

12. Koenen, K. C., Ratanatharathorn, A., Ng, L., McLaughlin, K. A., Bromet, E. J., Stein, D. J., … Kessler, R. C. (2017). Posttraumatic stress disorder in the world mental health surveys. *Psychological Medicine, 47*(13), 2260–2274. https://doi.org/10.1017/S0033291717000708

13. American Psychological Association (APA). (2017). *Ethical principles of psychologists and code of conduct.* https://www.apa.org/ethics/code/ethics-code-2017.pdf

14. Palmer, G. L. (2022). Using a Revolutionary Conscious Praxis (RCP) to Dismantle the Code of Silence as *Internalized Colonialism*. *Global Journal of Community Psychology Practice, 13*(1). https://doi.org/10.17161/gjcpp.v13i1.20627

15. Raypole, C. (2019). *30 grounding techniques to quiet distressing thoughts.* Healthline. https://www.healthline.com/health/grounding-techniques#mental-techniques

CHAPTER 1

I'll Beat the Black Off of You

Adverse Childhood Experience—Physical Abuse:

Physical abuse is when a parent, stepparent, or adult in the home intentionally harms a child through physical contact: pushing, grabbing, slapping, throwing something at the child, and hitting the child so hard that they are injured or have marks.[1]

THE RHYTHMIC TAPPING of raindrops on the window of my cozy private practice office created a soothing background as Mia settled deeper into the worn oversized chair across from mine. I sat, one leg crossed over the other, in patient observation, waiting for her to continue.

"It's like I let everyone down," Mia went on, her voice heavy with a mixture of what sounded like regret and frustration. "I'm supposed to be strong, the Fire Captain who could handle anything. And now … now I can't even control my own body."

Mia, a 51-year-old single Black female, had served as a dedicated firefighter for 26 years until a severe fall from a ladder forced her into an unexpected early retirement. She'd endured multiple surgeries over six months, yet the incident left her with a permanent physical impairment of her left leg and chronic pain. She was referred to my psychology practice at the university where I also taught through her worker's compensation benefits. Mia was seeking support for mood issues stemming from this chronic disability. After an intake and three therapy sessions, Mia was beginning to explore her emotions in depth.

"From what you've told me, it's understandable that you'd feel that way, Mia. You've carried a heavy burden of expectations for a long time, an expectation of strength for one. You're experiencing a great deal of physical pain right now and that's a lot for anyone to deal with long-term," I offered.

(dis)Honor Thy Mother: Daughterhood, Dysfunction and Deliverance, First Edition. Bridgette Peteet.
© 2026 John Wiley & Sons, Inc. Published 2026 by John Wiley & Sons, Inc.

"I haven't had pain like this since …" Mia hesitated.

I paused with her, knowing that silence can be a powerful tool in therapy, bridging paths to new exploration and insights.

"… since, my mother yanked my shoulder out of its socket when I was little," Mia continued.

The session had turned one way while my stomach turned another. Child abuse, past or present, spikes a defensive nerve in me, an urge to protect and defend. It's the reason why I treat adult clients and teach adult learners. Working with children weighs too heavily on my psyche. Back when I was an early trainee, it pained me to work with kids only to send them home to chaotic environments and abusive parents. There's constant mandated reporting, which requires psychologists and other health professionals to contact protective services for any suspicion of child or elder abuse or neglect. God bless those who have the stomach for child therapy because even after 20 years I do not.

Mia had already shared that her mother was deceased, and I was relieved, as a mandated reporter, not to have to investigate her mother's current access to and abuse of other children. Mia continued her story.

"I was six years old and roughhousing in the living room with my younger brother. He kicked over a table lamp and it shattered. I hurried to clean up the broken pieces but knew it was too late. Mom had heard. She was rushing toward me from the kitchen, not asking questions and yanking me up from the floor by my arm. I heard a loud pop. The pain was so unbearable that I fainted. From there, my memory fades. There was a surgery and there was a story."

"A story?"

"Yes. I can recall my mom, stepdad, and grandma at my hospital bedside after surgery telling me to say that I fell. They didn't want Mom to get into trouble. She'd been in jail before, and I didn't want to be the one to send her back. I was scared," Mia said tearfully.

"I've never told anyone that before," she finished just above a whisper.

"Well, I want to thank you for your vulnerability with me here today. How do you feel after sharing your story for the first time?" I probed gently.

"I feel free like a weight has been lifted. But also, a little bit guilty like I betrayed my mother by telling you. Looking back, I think my mother was mentally ill. She'd have these uncontrollable mood swings at times, hit me, and call me names. She could be very loving though. I know she loved me in her own way."

"It sounds like your mother may have certainly suffered from mental health issues; however, that doesn't absolve her from her parental responsibilities. It also doesn't erase the harm that was done to you. I think of these external forces like mental illness and substance abuse as explanations, not justifications. An explanation tells us why; it's a point of fact. Justification implies that an action is right, okay, or acceptable. Does that make sense to you Mia?"

"I never thought about it that way Doc. I've always blamed myself, made excuses for my mother, and been the dutiful daughter even until her death. I worked hard to make something of my life to please her. I think I might want to talk about that a bit more in here if that's okay."

"Yes, of course it is."

"I'm an expert in this," I thought silently.

I provided brief psychoeducation on adverse childhood experiences (ACEs) before summarizing our session and giving Mia the link to the ACEs questionnaire to complete before our next session.

Instead of immediately typing up my session note, I stared out the water-speckled window of the office high-rise. How many times had I treated "Mia"? Too many to count. It wasn't always a case of physical abuse; sometimes it was the hypercritical, excessively negative, or emotionally abusive mothers whose broken daughters ended up on my couch. How long would they suffer in silence? Something about that question felt hypocritical though. I'd never fully shared my story, even with my therapists. Maybe someday sharing my experience could help others, I thought. Memories began swirling like the thunderclouds above, dredging up my dark past to the surface.

***

The evening sun cast a faint glow on the quiet suburban street while shadows danced beneath the swaying trees. In one of the old paneled houses, behind a façade of normalcy, a different kind of storm brewed.

I was halfway up the carpeted staircase of my childhood home when her words struck me like a sudden gust. Swiveling on my heel, I gazed downward at my mother, Debra, who was springing up from the bathroom floor. The weight of regret settled in me instantaneously due to the unkind words I had only moments ago uttered to my younger sister, Devon.

Mom screamed at me, "THAT'S IT; I'VE HAD IT WITH YOU!"

Her tone carried a chilling promise—she was literally going to kill me this time. She ordered me back down the stairs, cussing and screaming at me the whole way. In the living room, she retrieved the 3-ft-long brown extension cord from the wooden corner cabinet, folding it in half with the ends in her grip. I hoped she'd hold on tight this time, or the pain and bruising from the stiff metal prongs or plastic inlet would make it doubly unbearable.

"I am going to beat the black off of you!" she promised.

My three siblings had hastily escaped to the next room, afraid of catching an accidental blow from an uncontrolled backswing. If they inadvertently got hit, she'd say it was for something else they had done that she didn't know about; there was never an apology.

I'd weighed the gravity of my crime, determining if I got to keep my clothing on as a mild buffer to the blows of the malleable plastic whip or whether I'd have to strip down to my bare skin. Jeans were the optimal shield, the only item that prevented welts. Sweatpants or khakis were equal, both lessening the sting of rubber meeting flesh. Shorts left the back of your lower legs exposed. My mother loved to show off her legs with smooth, light skin. At home, she usually wore shorts and let her breasts sag under her t-shirt in adult rebellion against her mother's strict rule to wear a "brassiere" 24/7. I was momentarily grateful that my legs were covered by slacks that day.

I trembled at Mom's approach, hands out in front in a defensive posture in case she struck early. Eyes blazing, she walked toward me and commanded, "Drop your pants!" My eyes widened in disbelief. I had misjudged my sentence. My older brother, Tony Jr., had been whipped nude for stealing money from Mom's purse or riding his bike to another city with friends in the middle of the night. That day, I'd voiced three little words to Devon.

I slowly complied with her command and unbuttoned my pants. I was an obedient child and had spent my life trying to avoid triggering her rage. If I did everything right, I hoped I wouldn't be beaten. But I still regularly miscalculated. I'd try to avoid the whippings my siblings got for things like skipping chores, poor grades, and fighting. Still, I'd find myself as the oldest daughter held equally responsible for their failure to complete an assigned task or not making them do their homework and got whipped, too.

In our family ecosystem, I was the responsible child and yet the scapegoat for our family problems. Tony was the designated golden child, the only boy and the oldest. He did little to earn this honor yet could do no wrong. Devon, the funny one, was the family mascot. Tanya was a toddler, and we didn't know yet what her appointed role would be. The toxic family roles were predictable and kept us fighting each other rather than joining forces against a common enemy.

I carefully slid my pants down my pubescent thighs, wishing my shirt was longer and covered my bottom. My face was wet from hot tears, snot, and saliva in anticipation of what was to come, but knowing that if I paused too long, it would only enrage Mom more. I reluctantly pushed my slacks to my calves and turned toward the sofa, offering my caramel backside.

The agony of the first blow shot through my body like a burning hot knife, instantly zapping me out of clear consciousness as I fell face-first onto the faded mauve couch. There was a distinct protocol when being whipped. No matter how much your back, butt, and legs stung or how much you believed you could not take anymore, you must still follow these rules.

Rule #1: Don't turn over onto your back. Turning over meant access to more vulnerable parts of your body, the parts not toughened by years of whippings. If struck, it would not stop the beating.

Rule #2: Never raise your arm above your head to protect yourself. She might take this gesture as a sign of aggression. You have to be a passive recipient and never hint at self-defense.

Rule #3 was the most important. Never, never, ever, ever, ever grab the bat, broom, belt, or cord as it is striking you. Not even by accident. A reflexive defensive movement to protect yourself could be misinterpreted as a threat, a defensive act against a parent, and the ultimate sign of disrespect.

Violating these rules would extend the beating and justify any fatality incurred.

As a perpetual rule follower, I did the only thing I could do. I dropped my body from the couch to the ground, squirming under each strike and screaming in agony.

When Tony Jr. got beat, he sometimes tried to show his bravery by holding his cries in for as long as he could. At 16, he'd perfected it. He had learned by then that men, especially Black men, were supposed to repress their emotions and avoid showing signs of weakness. But girls weren't judged in the same way. I was free to scream. So, I did.

I hoped my yells would reach my mother's heart. I wanted my cries to find our neighbor's ears. I wished that Mom would stop, that someone would stop her, that someone would save me.

Mom didn't hear me and didn't seem to worry about anyone else hearing me. If anyone else overheard my cries, they didn't come. They didn't call anyone to help either. Not at first. In the aftermath, Pawpaw came. In the following months, the authorities. For now, the only thing that came were more blows.

I counted her lashes as Mom continued to scream and swing at me. My adopted uncle/cousin, Juan, used to negotiate with Granny and Pawpaw about how many "licks" he would get before a punishment. If the answer was three, he felt he could stand it. But, five immediately sent him into despair.

I anticipated the end of Mom's attack, counting the strikes that matched the syllables of her words. Ever on beat, she'd swing, one "I'M" … two "SICK" … three "OF" … four "YOUR" … five "SH*T!"

That was higher than I had ever managed to count during one of her tirades. Mom had passed five and was still swinging. I was crying hysterically, screaming, turning, and twisting on the filthy floor, trying to offer her any unscathed piece of my flesh. I was senseless and beginning to crack.

My only escape might be fatigue setting in on Mom's 5′2″, round frame as she swapped the angles of her blows to cover my body in lashes and switched the weapon to a fresh hand. At 14, I was much taller than her but skinny, still waiting for curves to emerge in my late-developing body. I see portions of her face when I peek in the mirror; one passed down three generations from her mother to her, then me, and slimmed by my father's features. I accept or deny this fact depending on my internal strength that day. I am confident Mom saw herself and our father in me as she hovered over my defenseless frame, hating both reflections in my eyes.

There is a moment in a beating where your scream is lost in the throes of your gasps for breath, the sound and gestures out of sync, like the wind is knocked out of you. Your mouth motions to form a sound, but nothing comes out. Or, you are silenced by the certainty that your scream will be met with a threat not to scream lest you really "get something to cry about." Those who tried not to cry got beat longer, and those who screamed were told to SHUT UP!

In the 1980s and 1990s, corporal punishment was commonly the order of the day, particularly in Black families.[2] Before insights about the potential harm grew, attitudes shifted, and the law intervened, many families held firm to the belief that physical discipline was integral to raising resilient and respectful children. Today, the definition has evolved significantly. Any act that causes bodily injury to a child is a reportable criminal offense. Often drawing from their upbringing, some parents see whippings as a means to protect their children from potential harm and to keep them on the "straight and narrow." However, other parents struggle with stress and anger and sometimes used violence to unleash their frustrations.

My mind whirled out of control.

Why does she hate me? Why does my mother hate me?

But that was impossible. Mothers don't hate their daughters. They love their daughters unconditionally. Mothers are self-sacrificing and put their children first. Mothers provide security and trust and help children build their self-worth. That is what we're told.

Still, Mom's response was disproportionate to the punishment for a common retort lobbed at her annoying younger sister. It felt personal, and precisely because of what she'd said, she was sick of me. I had lit a match in her powder keg, and nothing could contain it.

My mind and body were straining to separate as if I were disassociating or worse, dying. I hovered above myself momentarily, watching in astonishment as my body convulsed on the floor—that poor girl. You could say I felt sorry for her. Because if it was happening to her, my mind could let me believe it wasn't happening to me. If I just thought hard enough, I could sit the pain over there with her and pretend that my real life was better. No one was hitting me over here in my imaginary world. There, my "real Mom" loved me. I'd tried this mental escape in my daydreams and was unsuccessful, but here, while trying to break free of excruciating pain, it felt like it might work. Run. Mental freedom from the pain was within reach, getting closer. My mind felt like it was pulling too far away from my body, but some surfacing part of me thought that was a terrible idea. That part was a life jacket. The tiny voice grew louder. I refused to sink under the wave of disconnection. I held on, kicking to the surface, and burst through with one last breath, sound, and voice joining back together. My mind and body reconnected at the same time. I had my mind. I needed my mind.

My mind had saved me. My mind would continue to save me. Something deep inside had pulled the two parts back together, mind and body. I held each piece with a death grip. I was silent, but my inner voice was growing loud. *Never again.*

Mom continued to let her verbal tirade rain down on me as I lay convulsing in pain on the dirty carpet. She was incensed about the self-inflicted lashes she'd acquired on the backswing of her haphazard strokes.

"LOOK WHAT YOU MADE ME DO!"

She twisted her arm to reveal two tiny red lines brushed across her beige skin. She struck me one last time for good measure, dropping the cord on my body this time. She stomped off toward the stairs, leaving me lying and quaking on the ground.

My siblings and I didn't usually help each other after a whipping. Then again, none of us had ever experienced anything as severe as what I'd just gone through. Tony and Devon, ages 16 and 12, flanked me, the middle child, and helped me to my feet. My baby, my sister Tanya, age 2, just cried. Among my older siblings, there was no smirk of satisfaction that occasionally accompanied a sibling's demise, a feeling of gratitude that it wasn't you. This time was different.

Together, they lifted me from the floor by my underarms, careful not to touch the burning, bleeding wounds covering my arms and legs. They guided me to the bathroom and propped me atop the toilet seat. We were well-versed in basic first aid because Mom had been a medical assistant and made us tend to our wounds with no empathetic words or kisses for our "boo-boos." My siblings moistened a clean washcloth and gently dabbed the cool liquid on the lesions on my skin before applying salve and dressing the most severe areas. It felt tremendous and horrendous at the same time. They helped me upstairs to my room and into my bed, where I couldn't stop crying from the physical and emotional pain. My body continued to convulse uncontrollably until it rocked me to sleep.

Someone had called our de facto 911 emergency contacts and saviors, Granny and Pawpaw, my mother's parents. Sometime that evening, when my spasms had finally ceased, I went outside to meet Pawpaw as he pulled his green conversion van in front of the house. I was too scared to talk to him inside lest Mom hear me "telling on her."

Pawpaw was the only one who could control Mom. He'd let her go on and on, too far for our liking, until he got fed up and halted her in her tracks with a stern "DEBRA!" She'd stop talking instantly. It was like magic, a spell we wished he would use more often.

Pawpaw was there now and I was momentarily vindicated. My hero was coming to save me. After all, as the eldest granddaughter, I was "Pawpaw's girl." I rushed out to the sidewalk as he swaggered around the corner from the driver's side.

I tattled about how Mom had beaten me unclothed while lifting bandages and modeling the lacerations on my arms and legs. More than 20 wounds ranged from short, slightly puffy welts to a 12-in. ridge winding down the back of my right thigh. Carefully, I lifted the gauze on the side of my bulging left wrist to reveal the most severe injury. I winced as the cloth detached, centimeter-by-centimeter, from the wide, burning u-shaped gash. My eyes watered either at the physical pain or the memory of being hit, I wasn't sure which.

Pawpaw was a man of few words, but his nonverbal language was loud.

Hmph!

It was his usual retort when he was moderately displeased. He'd been leaning down to see the scars on the bottom half of my body. He stood up straight when he finished his assessment.

"What did you do?"

Tears resurfaced in the inner corners of my eyes. I knew it was emotional hurt this time. I shook my head in disbelief that Pawpaw would ask me such a thing. I thought that the beating from Mom had been a clear violation of the unwritten code of discipline. Controlled, counted lashes commensurate with the severity of the problem behavior were culturally acceptable. Outliers were supposed to bring the family's wrath and consequences if you went too far. I would've been satisfied with a strong chastising or, at minimum, a passive comment to help Mom realize she was wrong. But this, this question, blamed me.

I can still remember Pawpaw standing there waiting for me to answer. I wanted to ask him, "Does it matter?" with a sassy shake of my neck but I wasn't crazy. Overt disrespect to an elder was an immediate death sentence. Instead, I obediently answered him. He would then certainly see that Mom was wrong and I hadn't broken the "rules" of the parent–child hierarchy.

"Mom told me to do Devon's chores, and I told Devon, 'I hate you.' "

In retrospect, I admit that it was displaced anger. Displacement is a psychological defense mechanism that involves redirecting one's emotional feelings or impulses from one's original source to a different, often less threatening target.[3] I was expressing hatred toward my mother through my sister, a safer outlet. Meanwhile, Mom was acting out. Acting out is another psychological defense mechanism characterized by expressing inner conflicts, emotions, or frustrations through disruptive or impulsive behaviors rather than verbal communication or introspection.[4] Of course, I wasn't attuned to any of that at 15.

After my brief story, Pawpaw was silent. That meant, on a basic level, he wasn't pleased. However, he didn't move to fault Mom either. I went on, making sure he understood the full risks at hand.

"And, I have to wear my cheerleading uniform to school tomorrow," I said self-righteously.

I shared this, knowing that if anyone at school saw my injuries, Mom might get in trouble. The smug part of me wanted someone to see. She was wrong, but someone else would have to say it. I had no more room for silent consent, indirectly defending and protecting Mom by hiding my scars.

"Can't you just wear leggings," Pawpaw offered with finality.

It was a cover-up, literally and figuratively. Cover up your scars and pretend nothing happened. Protect the adult, not the child. The event would be filed safely into the vault of family secrets. That vault, teeming at the seams, could hold no more. It would soon burst. Someone would be bold enough to make that anonymous, life-changing call. Someone would protect the children.

At school the next day, I pretended. I pretended that I wasn't in pain every time I slid into a hard, plastic desk seat. I faked forgetfulness that the team had agreed not to wear leggings with our uniforms. I couldn't get away with it at the football game, so I feigned generosity and let another girl "practice" being Captain. I went through the motions of cheering from the second row, careful not to turn my back toward the crowd. The top half of my body went through the motions of high and low V's at 40%, while my lower body kept still to avoid stretching my burning skin.

Fire it up, up
Everybody fire it up.
Fire it up, up
Everybody fire it up.

I put on a fake smile and mumbled through the short cheer, silently daydreaming of my escape from hell.

References

1. Centers for Disease Control (CDC). (n.d.). *Fast facts: Preventing adverse childhood experiences.* https://www.cdc.gov/violenceprevention/aces/fastfact.html
2. Gershoff, E. T., & Grogan-Kaylor, A. (2016). Race as a moderator of associations between spanking and child outcomes. *Family Relations, 65*(3), 490–501.
3. American Psychological Association (APA). (2023). *Displacement. American psychological association dictionary of psychology.* https://dictionary.apa.org/displacement
4. American Psychological Association (APA). (2018). *Acting out. American psychological association dictionary of psychology.* https://dictionary.apa.org/acting-out

CHAPTER 2

Some People Get Dealt All the Aces in Life

—Anne Mallory

Categories of Adverse Childhood Experiences[1]			
Abuse	*Neglect*	*Household Dysfunction*	
Physical Abuse	Physical Neglect	Mental Illness	Incarcerated Relative
Emotional Abuse	Emotional Neglect	Mother Treated Violently	Substance Abuse
Sexual Abuse		Divorce	

I AM A child abuse statistic. As I mentioned, I am also a licensed clinical psychologist. In combination, my profession has given me the language to name the abuse, failed systems, and suffering my siblings and I endured. Physical abuse is one type of childhood trauma called *adverse childhood experiences* (*ACEs*). Originally, there were ten.

I have taken ACEs training, read about it, supervised a dissertation, and published a paper on the topic. So, while I know the topic well, I do not consider myself an expert on ACEs research. On a personal level, I am a specialist, a master, a virtuoso, if you will, on the lived experience of ACEs. I have also worked with and supervised countless clinical cases with adults who experienced these types of childhood adversities. In particular, I have worked with dozens of women, especially Black women, who were abused by their mothers in similar ways and held their secrets shared within the safety of a confidential therapy room. I sit on the edge of my seat, trying to restrain myself from blurting out, "Girl, me too!" The sessions are about my clients, and it is not the time for me to process my traumas. I've had therapy for that, but it was eye-opening that I wasn't alone.

(dis)Honor Thy Mother: Daughterhood, Dysfunction and Deliverance, First Edition. Bridgette Peteet.
© 2026 John Wiley & Sons, Inc. Published 2026 by John Wiley & Sons, Inc.

Sadly, these women also feel like no one relates to their stories. They experience shame for "telling" on their mothers and a sense of betrayal for violating the cultural taboos of secrecy. They quickly backpedal and conceal their revelations with a counternarrative of gratitude, respect, and unconditional love for their mothers.

I silently resist transferring my emotions onto these clients, a process called countertransference,[1] avoiding a push for them to immediately tell their stories without the minimizers and masks of maternal redemption. But, a good clinician keeps me from pressing my agenda. I meet my patients where they are, help move them toward their desired treatment goals, and live past their trauma.

Mental health professionals have organized early traumatic experiences under an umbrella term called *ACEs*. ACEs include certain types of abusive events that occurred before the age of 18. The Center for Disease Control Kaiser Study initially recognized 10 ACEs, which include physical, emotional, and sexual abuse, physical or emotional neglect, and household dysfunction.[2] Over time, the list has expanded to include other adverse community experiences such as bullying, neighborhood safety, and racism[3,4] that I exclude in this book for brevity and because they occur outside the purview of immediate parental responsibility or oversight.

Most people (about 64%) in the United States have experienced one ACE.[5] Divorce is the most prevalent. Having one ACE increases the odds of having multiple. Those with three or more ACEs are less than 20% of the population. Between 1/6 and 1/8 (12.5–16.6%) of adults have four or more ACEs.[5] That is where the data stop, but I have eight.

That's *8 out of 10*.
That's *80%* of these childhood traumas.
That's *four-fifths* of the significant types of abuse.

There are more than 20,000 journal articles on ACEs. I haven't read them all, but I have noticed a pattern. The studies often consider everyone with four or more as one group.[2,6] At the de facto cut point of four, the consequences start to get serious as early childhood adversity has a dose relationship with serious health challenges in adulthood. Individuals with ACE scores of 4 or more were 12 times more likely to have attempted suicide, 7 times more likely to be alcoholic, and 10 times more likely to have injected street drugs. People with ACE scores of 6 and higher have an almost 20-year shortening of lifespan.[2] The consensus in the field seems to be that the prognosis is equally poor after four experiences and that having higher levels of adversity doesn't make it worse. Or perhaps there are just not enough of us with 5, 6, 7, 8, 9, or 10 ACEs to properly study what happens to us.

This gap makes it challenging to calculate how much of a "statistic" we might be. Following the empirical pattern that the data suggests, with eight ACEs, at best, I represent 2% of the population. I am what we call an outlier.[7] If accurate, it means that I have experienced more childhood trauma than 98% of the population in the United States. As I think about it, that number is shocking in the context of my childhood traumas, but even more so when I consider that I am an outlier in another regard, too.

As a child, the phrase "Don't be a statistic" had stuck in my head. Was it a part of a public service announcement? I don't remember where I heard it, but I understood it to mean avoiding crime, drugs, teen pregnancy, and other ills. The primary way I avoided these perils was to focus on school. I did *all* the school. While doing athletics, extracurriculars, and part-time jobs, I graduated high school in the top 10% of my class. I earned my bachelor's, master's, and doctorate over the next nine years. Earning a terminal degree, a PhD, put me among 2% of the population with this degree.[8] There it was again, 2%.

Crudely combining the two extremes of my life, I am 2% of 2% or 0.0004% of the population. I am an outlier in two opposing directions, ACEs at one end and education at the other. This places me in the exceptionally rare position to be able to comment on both the lived experience of ACEs, structural failures, and the underlying psychological factors associated with them.

The ACEs survey identifies the presence or absence of an experience in each category to get a total score. Research has found that this alone is useful for generally summarizing childhood trauma and predicting outcomes in adulthood. The results can help guide clinicians toward areas for follow-up and can inform recommendations for appropriate resources. However, the insiders (me and other survivors) and outsiders (clinicians and scientists) plainly understand that not all ACEs are created equal.[9] For example, experiencing a parental divorce, a typical ACE, may not be similar in severity to physical abuse. Furthermore, ACE scores tell us little or nothing about how severe the incidents were and how often, how many times, or when the abuse occurred.

These experiences are assessed retrospectively, meaning that the assessment relies on our flawed human memory. Even more, though every item asks about the involvement of the parents, family, or household members, these key figures are almost always ignored in the follow-up discussion, instead focusing on system failures and solutions. While valid, empathetic, and appropriate, this may minimize personal responsibility and relationship outcomes.

Despite its imperfections, this fantastic body of research consistently finds that higher numbers lead to higher consequences; specifically, as the number of ACEs increases, so do the negative outcomes. However, this relationship is not always direct.

Based solely on my score, I should be a mentally ill, physically unhealthy substance user who dropped out of school and has about 13 years to live. But I am not. I am not one of those things … well, maybe somewhat physically unhealthy thanks to perimenopause, and who knows about my life expectancy, but I digress. These were more accessible paths to avoid partly because I adopted an early plan to do the opposite of what I observed around me. The slogans of the 1990s helped, "Stay in School," "Just Say No," and "True Love Waits." By outward measures, I was killing it. I was in control (more like control issues, but I'd learn that about myself later).

We must also consider other outcomes, or what I like to call subclinical dysfunctions, which are symptoms or problems that are not severe enough to meet the psychological definitions of impairment. These maladjustments may include feeling like an impostor, people-pleasing, and tolerating emotional and physical abuse, abandonment issues, hypersensitivity, or a chronic need to prove oneself.[10,11] Many of us are unaware of these issues because they are less noticeable. We may or may not have linked these behaviors to our childhood trauma. Since it is less extreme, most individuals will never seek mental health treatment to address it. However, facing these issues will likely improve our emotional health, interpersonal relationships, and overall quality of life. This is the deep work of trauma recovery, and it can take a lifetime to root out and heal. We can't do it alone.

A solitary number fails to capture the entirety of who I am. Beyond that mere statistic, I wear various hats—a dedicated mother, a loving wife, a passionate volunteer, a cherished friend, a committed professor, and more.

As a mother, I take immense pride in my two remarkable teenage daughters, who excel academically, shine as athletes, and serve as leaders within their school. Objectively, I can proudly share that, despite my formative challenges, my daughters have thrived.

My husband, Damien, and I have nurtured our marriage for more than two decades. By "healthy," I don't mean perfect. There was a separation period when my daughters and I transitioned across the country. Damien had trouble finding employment in the West and the COVID-19 pandemic hit. That period was immeasurably stressful for families worldwide, but we ultimately reconciled and moved forward. We continue to share a deep commitment to our personal growth and the advancement of our family.

In addition to my roles within my family, I have healthy friendships and positive social outlets. I am interested in maintaining my physical health through diet, exercise, and sleep. I commit time to volunteering at my children's school and actively engage in community initiatives to improve citizens' health and close the achievement gap.

Becoming a psychologist was an unbelievable achievement that few anticipated, given my history and not what ACEs science would forecast. This accomplishment is resilient, immune to anyone's attempts to diminish it, even though I occasionally revisit a recurring dream where I must retake a high school class in my small-town hometown. This achievement holds exceptional significance for me, primarily because my pursuit of education in psychology served as an avenue to escape the adverse circumstances of my early life. It played a vital role in my healing process, allowing me to confront and recover from my childhood trauma and feelings of impostorism. Education provided a label for that trauma, validating my experiences and enabling me to unearth and rectify the cognitive distortions that once dominated my psyche, constantly whispering,

"You weigh too much."

"You're not street smart."

"You don't stand straight."

"You're not pretty."

"You don't enunciate enough."

"You are selfish."

"You are not compassionate enough."

"You are not strong enough."

"You are not enough."

That was the sum of it. No matter how hard I tried, I believed I would never be good enough … for her, my Mom. I was an impostor.

Neither my therapy nor the passage of time has fully quieted that "still small voice" of inadequacy. Faith tells me to listen because that voice should be God directing my life. Psychology informs me that hearing (audible) voices could be a sign of pathology. Nothing told me what to do when that voice originated from my mother.

I've said that a mother's words become a child's inner voice. There is no science to back this theory, but it was true for me. I'd made this connection in flashes of insight, but I wanted to step back and take stock of *what* happened to me as a child. More importantly, I wanted to focus on *who*.

I have seen and used the ACE instrument many times. When working with clients or patients, I have causally noted the items I would answer in the affirmative, but I had never taken the "yes/no" survey until writing this book. I needed to take full stock before embarking on this emotional endeavor. And then, suddenly, there it was in a large blue box in the center of my screen. Seeing that high number splayed across my computer monitor caused me to pause. A survey confirmed that I was not misjudging or exaggerating what had happened to me as a child. It was real, and the face directly or indirectly hovering behind each question was my mother.

References

1. American Psychological Association (APA). (2018). *Countertransference. APA dictionary of psychology.* https://dictionary.apa.org/countertransference

2. Felitti, V. J., Anda, R. F., Nordenberg, D., Williamson, D. F., Spitz, A. M., Edwards, V., … Marks, J. S. (1998). Relationship of childhood abuse and household dysfunction to many of the leading causes of death in adults: The Adverse Childhood Experiences (ACE) Study. *American Journal of Preventive Medicine, 14*(4), 245–258.

3. Harris, N. B., & Renschler, T. (2023). CYW adverse childhood experiences questionnaire – teen self-report. *Center for Youth Wellness.* https://centerforyouthwellness.org/wp-content/uploads/2018/06/CYW-ACE-Q-TEEN-SR-1-copy.pdf

4. Wade, R., Shea, J. A., Rubin, D., & Wood, J. (2014). Adverse childhood experiences of low-income urban youth. *Pediatrics, 134*(1), e13–e20. https://doi.org/10.1542/peds.2013-2475

5. Centers for Disease Control (CDC). (n.d.). *Fast facts: Preventing adverse childhood experiences.* https://www.cdc.gov/violenceprevention/aces/about.html#:~:text=ACEs%20are%20common%20across%20all,%2C%20learn%2C%20work%20and%20play.

6. Webster, E. M. (2022). The impact of adverse childhood experiences on health and development in young children. *Global Pediatric Health, 9,* 2333794X221078708. https://doi.org/10.1177/2333794X221078708

7. American Psychological Association (APA). (2018). *Outlier. APA dictionary of psychology.* https://dictionary.apa.org/outlier

8. World Population Review. (2025). *PhD percentage per country 2025.* https://worldpopulationreview.com/country-rankings/phd-percentage-by-country

9. Briggs, E. C., Amaya-Jackson, L., Putnam, K. T., & Putnam, F. W. (2021). All adverse childhood experiences are not equal: The contribution of synergy to adverse childhood experience scores. *The American Psychologist, 76*(2), 243–252. https://doi.org/10.1037/amp0000768

10. Gu, W., Zhao, Q., Yuan, C., Yi, Z., Zhao, M., & Wang, Z. (2022). Impact of adverse childhood experiences on the symptom severity of different mental disorders: A cross-diagnostic study. *General Psychiatry, 35*(2), e100741. https://doi.org/10.1136/gpsych-2021-100741

11. Yeo, G., Lansford, J. E., Hirshberg, M. J., & Tong, E. M. (2024). Associations of childhood adversity with emotional well-being and educational achievement: A review and meta-analysis. *Journal of Affective Disorders, 347*, 387–398.

CHAPTER 3

There's No Place Like Home

Adverse Childhood Experience—Emotional or Psychological Abuse:

Emotional abuse is any intentional act that harms a child's emotional well-being or self-worth. Examples of emotional abuse include: name-calling, shaming, rejection, withholding love, and threatening.[1]

IT WAS 2:57 P.M. one chilly fall afternoon in my high-rise office at the university. Engrossed in catching up on never-ending emails, I awaited my 3 o'clock appointment for academic advising. The student scheduled to meet with me was Josh, a familiar face from my senior-level Research Methods class the previous Spring semester. He had excelled in the course and was among the few who regularly used my office hours.

Over time, we'd developed a rapport as he'd shared the all-too-familiar struggles of being a first-generation college student. I'd been advising him in preparation for his graduate school admissions applications in psychology. Today, he sought assistance with his personal statement, arriving with a first draft that immediately raised concerns.

"I am a white, heterosexual, cisgender male."

Red flag. The admissions committee seeks a genuine understanding of applicants, and such statements, resembling a client's demographic profile, fall short of conveying a meaningful sense of cultural self-awareness.

"After a troubling childhood, at age 10, I was diagnosed with Obsessive Compulsive Disorder (OCD)."

Red flag. While transparency about personal struggles is becoming increasingly acceptable, it is crucial to strike a balance in presenting such information within the context of a competitive application process.

"The prior year, a social worker had come to my house and removed me from my parent's care due to our living conditions. That's why I want to become a psychologist, to help kids like me."

(dis)Honor Thy Mother: Daughterhood, Dysfunction and Deliverance, First Edition. Bridgette Peteet.
© 2026 John Wiley & Sons, Inc. Published 2026 by John Wiley & Sons, Inc.

Red flag and trigger. While the statement expresses a genuine desire to help others, it is important to approach this narrative with caution. Psychologists indeed work to support individuals facing various challenges, but the specific act of removing a child from their parents' care is typically within the purview of child protective services caseworkers, not psychologists.

Josh also had no idea that his story mirrored mine more than he could have imagined.

***

Spurred by an anonymous report, CPS and the police arrived unannounced like a SWAT team at our doorstep, tasked with conducting a child welfare assessment. Devon, a 12-year-old latchkey kid, was home alone after school and answered the door. Nervous at the presence of legal officials, she called our typical first responder, Granny. She sent back-up in the form of their youngest, 19-year-old daughter April. The CPS worker, a young white woman, asked Devon and April to show her around. The police officers remained outside. The county agent entered the house, with a clipboard and a pen in hand.

If cleanliness is next to godliness, the house was unholy. The foul stench of animal and human feces mingled in the air. Searching for the source in the front room, the woman found piles of dog feces behind the reclining chairs graying with dirt and dust. She kept walking and turned right toward the bathroom. She tried not to gag. Eyes watering, she checked the sink. There was no running water, but a red water cooler sat half-filled in the tub. She marked an X on her clipboard. The toilet overflowed with human excrement. Her nose likely burned. Inadequate plumbing, X.

She moved through the blanketed doorway, used to trap the heat from the hearth, and found herself in the living room, houseflies buzzing. The laundry room was immediately to her right, so she turned there first. In that 5 × 10 space, she saw the ceiling heaving and holed from the weight of water pouring in from the roof. A mountain of dirty, crusty clothes was piled as high as the top of the broken washer and dryer. X. She walked back into the living room to take a closer examination.

***

"Does this wood-burning stove work?" she asked Dev.

"Yes, but it leaves black soot in your nose," Dev shared. At least there was one source of heat. Check.

Off the living room, she stepped in the doorway of Tony's room with junk piled on top of a mattress almost to the ceiling. Tony usually just slept in the living room on the couch. X.

Cats scurried as the woman moved into the kitchen through the other draped doorway. She twisted the oven burner. Nothing happened. She regretted opening the refrigerator and releasing the stench into her tortured nostrils. She checked the cabinets and found an abundance of seasonings and little food. She also discovered the daytime commune of the cockroach community that resided within the depths. X X X.

Upstairs.

She slowly opened the first door on the right, finding a bedroom resembling a comfortable jail cell with carpet and a stiff yellow blanket atop a single twin bed. There had been a poor attempt to brighten the room with lavender paint that had splattered along the baseboards. To the woman's surprise, no clothes or trash were strewn around the floor. Crates had been converted into a 2 × 2 shelf. She took a momentary recess.

"Is this your mother's room?" she asked her tiny tour guide.

"No, it belongs to my older sister, Bridgette," Dev replied.

"It's the only clean room in the house," the agent let slip out, but Dev and my Aunt caught it.

Devon took offense. She'd just cleaned her room. She'd shoveled everything into the two-door closet, piling it to the ceiling. If you can't see it, it's clean—same thing. The social worker found Dev's hidden "treasure" when she progressed through her room next.

The woman finished her tour at the end of the hallway. The last bedroom. Clothes, shoes, blankets, food containers, and cups covered every surface, including the floor. It was the mother's room.

She carried her clipboard, heavy with X's marking the deficits in basic needs, back downstairs. She didn't know that there were even more problems that she hadn't found.

Outside, she pulled my aunt to the side.

"You need to call your sister. The kids are going to be removed immediately."

Dev packed many of her belongings and rode to Granny's house with my aunt. The social worker and her team followed them for the short distance.

They called my mother at work. She didn't answer. Granny offered to help. Legally, it had to be our father. They got ahold of him, and he came to pick us up.

The next day at school, I got called down to the office. I never got into trouble. I avoided trouble. It was a strange request. I strolled to the front of the building.

I entered through the glass-paned door, and the Vice Principal gave me a stare that conveyed kindness and sympathy. OK, I wasn't in trouble. She gestured for me to follow her, and I skulked behind her 6'2' frame toward the conference room.

I was relieved when I saw Tony Jr. sitting at the large table in the room. Across from him sat a young white woman wearing sensible beige slacks and a wrinkled dress shirt. She introduced herself. She was the social worker—the one who had been in our house and had upheaved us from our lives.

First at our home and now at school. What was coming next? I began to shut down in anger. I was humiliated. In my mind, everyone at school now knew what happened at home. I'd worked hard to keep my school and home life separate. I was a model student and was active in clubs and cheerleading. Her presence breached my façade. Intruder.

I flopped into the seat next to my brother, and she started asking us questions. Tony matched my anger, and I figured we could take her together. She wasn't going to hurt us any more than she already had. White people in our town usually backed down if we puffed up. They feared those of us from the "south side." It was the south side of a small town, but they didn't seem to know any better. Their response was always amusing because nothing dangerous happened in our rural community.

Instead of backing down, the social worker sidestepped our teenage anger.

"I can understand that you all are upset about being taken from the only home you've ever known. I'm sorry, but it's my job to ensure you all are safe," she shared calmly.

"Why did you come to the school? Now, everyone is going to know our business!" I retorted.

"The Vice Principal is the only person who knows why I am here."

Oh, okay. My defenses began to disarm. My anger evaporated, and guilt decided to take its turn.

I had failed to take care of the house. It was my fault. That's how Mom would see it. Yet, the social worker didn't ask me what I did or didn't do around the house. She didn't say what I should have or could have done. She'd even commended me for keeping my room tidy, doing well in school, and caring for my younger siblings. She finished her recap. Then, she leaned in and said as if reading my mind, "It's not your fault." It was one of the first times that I felt seen. And, for some reason, I believed her.

Reflecting on the past, I am grateful for the reassurance and the tangible step taken to remove us from that challenging physical environment. However, I am puzzled by the absence of inquiries into other forms of abuse we were enduring. While the relocation addressed our living conditions, it became evident that we needed more than just a change in surroundings. A comprehensive support system, encompassing various dimensions of our well-being, would have been beneficial. Targeted interventions to support our emotional and psychological health could have played a crucial role in fostering a more holistic recovery and resilience.

It was about a week before we saw our mother again. I fantasized about having a joyous reunion, perhaps sharing our abrupt separation's collective trauma. I'd been worried about her while we were away and was excited to see her. Mom did not feel the same.

Her face was set in a way that made her lower right jawbone protrude from her round face. She shrugged off our attempts to hug her. Hurt and dejected, we sat back down in Granny's living room and listened; silence was our only resistance.

"The filth in the house is your guys' fault!"

"I'm the cleanest person on the planet."

"I just gave up cleaning behind you nasty children."

"If you all had done your chores, I wouldn't be in this mess."

"Bridgette, you are older and should know better."

My mother's rejection and accusations did not land on me as they usually would, a rare moment that I did not beat myself up alongside her. I silently defended myself, armed with two facts. CPS had counted the squalor of my mother's bedroom among the rest of the ruins and had singled out my room as the exception. And the social worker's voice echoed in my ears, "It's not your fault."

Mom exhibited symptoms of a hoarding disorder characterized by persistent acquisition of possessions and a significant lack of insight into the severity of the condition.[2,3] Hoarding disorder affects 2–6% of adults.[4] This propensity for clutter likely stemmed from intergenerational transmission from Granny, born during the Great Depression, who clung to items like 36 laundry detergent scoops and decades-old JCPenney catalogs "just in case." While Granny was hygienic and organized with her possessions, meticulously cleaning daily and adhering to a ritualistic Friday housekeeping routine for Sabbath, she hoarded unnecessary items in hidden locations—bins, totes, and bags stored secretly in closets, under beds, and in the attic. Unlike Granny, Mom's hoarding was unhinged as recounted above, leading to significant consequences: legal intervention by CPS and repeated evictions.

Mom was nearing the end of her accusatory speech when she hit us with a whammy.

"We're moving to Columbus. I found a place." Her round eyes bulged, and her lips pursed.

The capital city of Ohio was 30 minutes away. It might as well have been the moon.

"It's closer to my job and will keep these rinky-dink small-town folks out of my business!"

I felt like I was drowning. I'd lived in Delaware my entire life. Mom had, too; heck, Granny had been born and raised here. We were country folk who knew nothing about the city. I was afraid that the schools weren't of the same caliber and that I would get bullied. I was terrified of her boyfriend, Ricky, who'd come to us straight from prison. Our safety net at Granny's house down the tracks would be ripped from under us. We began to protest.

Mom waved us off. "Y'all can still go to the same schools."

I tried to mask my doubt. She barely made sure Tony Jr. attended school as it was. My older brother was now behind me in the 9th grade and would eventually drop out. Mom had successfully clipped his wings ensuring that he would have to rely on her for the rest of his life. I had to do something before Mom ruined my life forever.

***

The previous summer, I had a respite staying at my grandparent's house to help them take care of two of my younger cousins while their parents were deployed in the Middle East. Granny and Pawpaw were strict and conservative, but their home was clean and stable. I considered moving to my dad's house for a moment, but I always felt like an intrusive houseguest there. It was exhausting trying to follow all of his rules—"Don't touch the wall"; "pick up that invisible crumb on the floor." He also lived in the boondocks. Granny's house was the better choice.

My grandparents agreed to the arrangement. There was only *one* condition. I'd have to be the one to tell my mother. They were her parents, but didn't want to deal with her.

I'd hoped they would at least join me in telling her. She'd only go so far out of pocket with her parents, especially her Dad. With me, Mom had few limits.

I thought it all through. Worst-case scenario, I'd get a beating like the one that had happened a year earlier. In the best-case scenario, Mom would scold me until I folded. I imagined the conversation would be like getting jumped *out* of a gang. I'd risk losing my life now to live a better life later. I reckoned she might not beat me with CPS still watching her, but I decided to tell her out in the open … just in case.

I had 1,462 reasons that I no longer wanted to live with Mom. Most of them were about her, but I couldn't say any of those things to her without immediately setting her off. I tried to think of everything she was going to say and do. I rehearsed it until the last possible minute.

Nearly a month later, we returned to that childhood home on a salvage mission to recover the remnants of our old life that we'd left behind in our hasty departure. We'd taken things over to Granny's house to store temporarily. We were finishing packing the last of our things in the trunk of Mom's old blue sedan. It was my last chance. It was now or never.

Mom liked to wear hospital scrubs when she wasn't working. It led people to ask her what she did for a living. She'd switched out the matching green top for an old white t-shirt and covered her short hair with a dark-blue moisture-zapping cotton bandana. Her bare face was greasy from the evening's labor. At Mom's insistence, we'd put in a little extra effort to destroy the house further. The mortgage was in her second husband William's name, likely a result of refinancing back when they were married. Mom wanted revenge. She would leave nothing for him to reclaim. She reached her goal. The house would eventually be condemned and demolished, taking the tormented walls holding our secrets to their grave.

Life as we knew it had been destroyed, our childhood home, our childhood. We were physically and emotionally displaced. Mom planned to move us to the city where I knew things were destined to get worse. I couldn't go. I wouldn't go. It was my last chance. If I was going to survive, I had to fight.

***

The sun was setting on our backs as my daughters and I hopped on our bikes after an afternoon at the park to make the one-mile trek down the trail toward home—this paved trail wound between suburban houses in a residential neighborhood. While my daughters and I couldn't be described as "outdoorsy" types, the COVID-19 pandemic kept us cooped up in the house for months. So, this simple bike ride marked a welcome break from our indoor confinement.

We'd stopped by the park and said hello to our only friends. "Only," b/c we didn't know anyone else. We'd moved across the country to California right before the pandemic—perfect timing. The playground was cordoned off with yellow caution tape, limiting the children to made-up games in the grassy areas. With the sun beginning its initial descent, it signaled that it was time for us to head back home.

Taryn, our eldest, assumed the lead down the path with preteen self-assurance. Jordyn, age 9, was positioned securely in the middle while I followed behind, watching our progress. We barely covered 50 ft when a massive tan cat emerged from the thickets and started crossing the trail directly ahead of us. This was no ordinary housecat.

The mountain lion, her shoulder muscles visibly rippling, pivoted her head in our direction as she gracefully moved across our path. Taryn wasted no time and swiftly began pedaling with all her might on her trusty Huffy bike. *Flight.*

Jordyn quickly dismounted her bike, her legs trembling as she stood rooted. *Freeze.*

Without hesitation, I leaped off my bike and hurried toward Jordyn, clutching my handlebars. My first impulse was to shield and protect her. *Fight.*

All I had to protect my child was a 20-lb, 10-speed bicycle. Quickly, I positioned Jordyn in a protective V-shape between our two bikes, angling the front wheel toward the untamed predator. The mountain lion had locked her gaze on us but continued striding toward the trail's opposite side, eventually breaking into a gentle jog.

"Get back on your bike! GO!" I shouted at Jordyn. Taryn was already shrinking in the distance, fleeing the scene. Without a second thought, we raced for home, our hearts pounding as if the lion were still in pursuit. Breathless and trembling, we finally arrived safely inside our garage five minutes later.

While motherhood certainly amplified it, I'd begin to grow into a fighter in my teenage years.

***

Outside in the driveway of our ramshackle childhood home, I turned toward Mom as we prepared to depart. I feigned casualness, but my insides were frozen in fear. I clenched my gut and shifted gears, preparing for the fight that was sure to come.

"Granny and Pawpaw said I could live with them," I yelled as if it were their idea and not mine. I figured they owed me at least that for not having this conversation with me. I also thought it might deflect some of Mom's anger toward them and not me. I was wrong.

Mom's mood shifted immediately. The air became thick, and it was hard to breathe.

"I am getting all A's in school, and I don't want to miss any days with the commute."

She replied, "I'll take you to school."

"But I have extracurriculars and games after school and need to live closer."

She latched on to that, thinking she'd won, conversation over.

"Mom and Dad would *never* let you cheer on Friday nights."

My grandparents agreed I could cheer if it did not disrupt their Sabbath. No calls. No rides. No, nothing on Friday nights. I also had to go to church with them every Saturday, even if I was tired, no questions asked.

"We already discussed it, and they said it was okay."

Mom had nothing. I'd passed Level 1 of the fight.

She moved from a defensive to an offensive position in a verbal attack. I listened enough not to risk being accused of ignoring her but with sufficiency to limit the penetration of her words. All I had to do was keep standing. Soundlessly, I hummed one of my favorite hymns,

I shall not, I shall not be moved
I shall not, I shall not be moved
Just like a tree planted by the water
I shall not be moved.

Mom went in.

"You're spoiled."

"You're selfish."

"You're abandoning your *real* family."

"Your little sisters need you."

Pulling my little sisters into the mix, I swayed a bit.

She was right, but still I could not go. Not even for them. I was fighting for my survival and would have to try to protect them from afar.

Her attack wasn't working, so she switched tactics again. She started to cry.

"Oh, so I must've been a *terrible* mother."

"Why don't you love me?"

"Why are my parents trying to take my children away from me?"

I tried to reassure her through my tears.

"You aren't a terrible mother," I lied.

"I do love you." The truth.

"I'm the one who asked to go. Please don't blame Granny and Pawpaw," I defended the adults.

I could tell that Mom wasn't listening to anything I was saying. She rolled her eyes and brushed off every retort of mine. She was going to make me go with her.

For a second, I visualized her forcing me into the car, me resisting by planting my feet against the doorframe. The only way I was going was by force. A new wave of resolve kicked in, and my back stiffened.

I whispered firmly, "I am not going."

She'd used every strategy short of putting her hands on me but had not won. Then, she made a countermove that I hadn't anticipated.

"If you go and live with your grandparents, you have to leave your dollhouse with me."

That day, I'd carefully carried the handmade wooden dollhouse my dad had built for me to the car. I planned to transport it safely on my lap instead of risking it getting smashed in the trunk. I'd been so careful with it over the years, keeping it displayed proudly on my dresser and fighting my sisters when they tried to force their oversized Barbies inside the petite cottage. It was my sole prized possession.

Thin brown wood framed the two-story home with a living room, a kitchen, and two bedrooms upstairs. I imagined that one was for me and my husband and the other was for a baby I wasn't sure I wanted, fearful that I was too wounded to ever parent. The plastic windows and front door mimicked the look of glass with white paint-etched designs in each. The window boxes and shutters replicated a real home. The backside was open, giving access to gentle play. I had a few pieces of furniture, a rocking chair, a kitchen table, and beds that I'd move around when "redecorating." My dad must have spent hours gluing together the wooden pieces. It was the most meaningful thing he'd ever done for me.

I'd often escape my real house into the imaginary middle-class world of my dollhouse. In it, I dreamed of my future, where my unborn kids were nurtured and loved. It meant everything to me. *Almost.*

"It'll be a symbol that you're still a part of our family," Mom continued with an insincere half-smile.

That dollhouse flashed before my eyes. That dollhouse would be demolished under her care as our real house would eventually be. I imagined it being decimated—piece by piece.

I saw the smugness on her face. She thought she'd won.

Then I whispered, "Okay."

Her face instantly soured. She'd made the mistake of setting the terms too low. Adulthood, only three years away, felt like an eternity. I had to get out now. It was my last chance. My eyes glinted in victory.

Irreverently, she took the dollhouse from the car's roof and put it in the backseat of her sedan. She lobbed a few more insults at me over her shoulder as she walked to the driver's side. None of them registered.

Like the social worker, I'd inspect the dollhouse each time I visited my mother's new place. Each time, a new portion was damaged. The window boxes were missing. X. The plastic on the front door was punched out. X. The walls were covered in magic marker graffiti. X. Eventually, the entire half of the roof was torn off. X.

I tried to make repairs, gluing back the broken pieces I found in my little sister's toy box, scraping off stickers, and begging them to leave it alone. It hurt less and less each time because I knew what to expect. By their second move, less than a year later, my dollhouse was utterly trashed. I almost shed a tear when I heard they'd thrown it into a dumpster. I didn't cry. It was worth it. Saving my life was far more critical.

The social worker had missed so many more Xs. Many other kinds of abuse were less pronounced or yet to come. She probably didn't want to know. What she could see had been enough. What she couldn't see, what others couldn't see, and what I could only partially see then was that it was so much more profound.

I'd physically escaped my mother. Mentally, I had a long way to go. Eventually, even that wouldn't be enough.

Leaving didn't end it. It just changed the scenery. Mom could let me go, but she couldn't let go of control. She would maintain it through guilt, confusion, lies, shame, isolation, or intimidation. One way or another, she'd find a way to hold power over me— an emotional hostage.

***

Mom paraded between her duplex's dining area and living room, pocket pistol cocked at a 90° angle. I was 19, and Mom had bought the tiny gun for "protection." Protection from what? I never knew. Not much happened on the "mean" streets of "Small Town, USA." Mom would bring the gun out to clean at odd times, usually in front of company. This time, her routine was for my college boyfriend. He sat anxiously as my mother talked more to herself than anyone else in the room.

"I'll bust a cap in his a$$."

Her threat was directed toward an imaginary assailant who got out of line or broke into her apartment. After her pretend shots, she'd blow make-believe smoke from the tip of the barrel. She might as well have said "bang, bang" for effect. I always watched her performance with a slight fear that someone would get hurt, but mostly in amusement at her child-like posturing.

Mom meant to threaten, manipulate, and intimidate those around her without ever pulling the trigger. We were too big to be beaten, but she'd found a new weapon. Her arsenal would continue to grow and evolve.

References

1. Centers for Disease Control and Prevention (CDC). (n.d.). *Fast facts: Preventing adverse childhood experiences.* https://www.cdc.gov/violenceprevention/aces/fastfact.html
2. American Psychiatric Association. (2022). *Diagnostic and statistical manual of mental disorders* (5th ed., text rev.). https://doi.org/10.1176/appi.books.9780890425787
3. Bratiotis, C., Muroff, J., & Lin, N. X. (2021). Hoarding disorder: Development in conceptualization, intervention, and evaluation. *Focus, 19*(4), 392–404.
4. Postlethwaite, A., Kellett, S., & Mataix-Cols, D. (2019). Prevalence of hoarding disorder: A systematic review and meta-analysis. *Journal of Affective Disorders, 256,* 309–316. https://doi.org/10.1016/j.jad.2019.06.003

CHAPTER 4

If I Was Such a Horrible Mother, How Did You Turn Out So Well?

Reflecting on Adverse Childhood Experiences

Reflecting on ACEs can be an overwhelming and painful process. The emotional weight of revisiting trauma, coupled with the fear of reliving pain or confronting unresolved feelings, makes this reflection difficult yet often beneficial for healing.[1]

GENTLY, WE DROVE through the sharp gravel, trying to avoid scraping the paint on the lower part of our car. It had been a two-hour drive, long enough to shake off the nerves I had felt since I'd received the invitation for this anticipated gathering.

"We must be at the wrong address," I quipped to my husband, Damien, as we pulled into an unmarked parking spot.

I eyed the building that looked more like a deserted horses' stable than a winery. I stared at its faded brown wood face and the white plastic lawn chairs scattered in front.

We paid $100 for this?

The nervousness resurfaced. Instantly, I felt out of place, though I was home.

I was back in Delaware, Ohio, a city with one public high school. The nearby Walmart put most of the retail shops in the historic downtown district out of business back in the day. The town had acquired a few new restaurants and shops in the 20 years since I'd moved away for college. There had never been much to do for entertainment, so I was impressed to hear that there was now a winery. I had visited wineries before in my travels. Most had a charming blend of rustic elegance. This one missed a part.

The parking lot boasted more pickup trucks than sedans, and one proudly displayed a Confederate flag bumper sticker. A short white man jumped down from the driver's seat of the one parked next to us. I peeked through our tinted windows at his familiar face.

Was it Nathan or Ryan? After all these years, I couldn't remember the names of most of my old classmates.

Nathan-Ryan wore a baseball cap, a white t-shirt under an open gray flannel, and faded blue jeans. Praying he was there for a different event, but knowing the truth, regret began to set in.

Mentally, I'd anticipated the high school reunions of Hollywood movies, a grand entrance into a dimly lit, music-filled ballroom, and everyone's shock at my "glow-up." I'd obsessed over finding the right outfit. I'd felt self-assured when I put on the fit and flare LBD (little black dress) with lace embroidery over a gold-paneled plunging V, giving the illusion of skin. My strappy black-and-gold high heels and clutch pulled the look together. As a bonus, the dress had pockets. I could hide my PhD in there. Not literally, but figuratively, like an ace card that I could whip out to end the anticipated comparison games that start with, "So what do you do for a living?" I'd selected a dark gray suit with a deep coral dress shirt and a complementing tie for my husband. He was cut, shaven, shiny, and ready for display. Go in or go home. It was now or never.

Spotting a pair of khakis and a casual dress on another couple entering the building gave me the confidence boost I needed. We came all this way. We might as well do it.

"Let's just go in," I suggested to Damien, thinking maybe it was better inside.

Damien pushed through the swinging wood door, and we stopped short in the bright light of the narrow diner-like room. Booths lined the walls on the left, with 4-seaters down the middle. I thought we were in a lobby for a moment, but the other doors had distinct labels, "restrooms" and "kitchen." I could smell our dinner as it sat atop the wooden bar in a row of foil chafing dishes, wafting a scent more like cafeteria-grade rigatoni than fine dining. Next to it sat a plastic dispenser of red mystery punch.

Fifty or so people clustered in small groups near the door. I grinned back at a few vaguely familiar eyes that had looked in our direction when we walked into the room. There were no brown faces or others I would have called friends. We moved awkwardly through the crowd, happily relinquishing our stage to the next victim who entered.

A pregnant belly pushed its way through the crowd toward us. The owner of that abdomen had her blonde hair pulled up and her blue eyes set on me. The distinct toothy smile gave her away. It was my old high school friend and college roommate, Elizabeth. She pulled me into a tight hug, and some of the tension in my stomach released. I introduced her to my husband. She beamed up at him and offered a polite greeting.

"Nice!" she whispered in my ear.

She steered us toward the group of tables where she'd been sitting before her rescue mission. A good-sized group had gathered. Most of them had familiar faces or names or were the partners of these acquaintances. Elizabeth introduced or reintroduced us to everyone. With a twinkle of pride, she added that she couldn't believe her old roommate was a doctor.

Her proclamation was as awkward as our fancy outfits. Elizabeth was a teacher, but it seemed as if few others had ever finished college. The kids who had been in honors classes with me were now professional dog walkers and sales representatives. Over the years, I'd run into a few who had dropped out of college—servers at restaurants and hotel workers who pretended not to know me when I visited. I hadn't known it was a theme.

"A PhD. Wow!" Elizabeth repeated, too loudly for my comfort.

Most around the table were not quick enough to stop their microexpressions as shock or humility crossed their faces, perhaps revealing their true feelings.[2,3] This had not been the plan. This educational weapon had been solely reserved for my past haters—people like the boy in Honors English who responded to my career essay about my dreams of becoming a lawyer with, "The only thing I can see you being is a secretary." I was saving it for the class mean girl, Emily, who'd exclaimed things like, "My daddy said the only reason you made cheerleading and I *didn't* is because they had to have a Black girl," and "Girls who weigh more than 125 lbs are fat. No offense," while being two sizes larger than me.

We ate cheap lasagna and talked awkwardly, catching up on the town's gossip until someone brought out a stack of yearbooks from our freshman through senior years. I was familiar with the photos from two of the books I'd purchased in the last year of middle and high school. Those were satisfactory, nothing to be too embarrassed about. I'd never seen the three books in between.

My husband flipped to the freshman section near the front of the second yearbook. Scrolling to the M's, he burst out in an uncontrollable, whole-body, knee-slapping whoop. He turned the book toward me. We'd generally chuckle *with* each other at these sorts of things, but I was silent as I took in the photo. Others looked over my shoulder, wanting in on the joke but politely staying quiet.

I stared at the familiar yet unfamiliar girl in the one-inch black-and-white photo. Her thin, greasy face tilted toward the right of the frame. Her eyes were squinting more than looking since she'd removed her glasses to improve the picture. She held her full lips together in a slight grin, covering her overbite and hiding the depth of her dimples. Her short, "middle school" hair was coarse on the bottom with straightened ends bent in a slight wave. She'd combed it lazily off to the side and backward, revealing a prominent widow's peak on her diminutive forehead. The no-name turtleneck sweater showed her shoulders, not helping or hurting the pain-filled image.

For a second, the live and still images merged. There was a glimmer of the woman today deep behind the forced grin of the young girl. She had big ideas for herself and would one day appreciate the full power of positive visualization. She looked into the future and could envision herself as a professional clad in a tailored skirt suit and crisp blouse. She'd never get "too big for her britches" and overpay for excessive designer shoes and handbags, anchoring herself in a history of poverty and pain while reaping some of the benefits of the middle class. She welcomed a time when her hair would be professionally maintained in slender locks curled to her waist, often mistaken for weave. Hair that would become her distinguishing feature rooted in appreciation of her heritage and representative of the health and healing she'd acquire. She'd balance her career and family, ensuring her children's every need was met. Her husband had no face back then, but she vowed that unlike her mother there would only be one. She'd be assertive and confident. That girl had dreams. That girl would show her strength, courage, and independence soon. She would no longer be an imposter. She'd find her voice.

Silently, I whispered to her. *You're going to be alright.*

I closed the book.

We said our goodbyes rather than farewells, knowing thankfully that we'd never see my former classmates ever again. We crossed back through the parking lot, with fancy black shoes covered in dust and matching the mud flaps on the row of pickup trucks that lined our way.

My mind wandered. I used to love pickup trucks but over time something changed. My dad, Tony, Sr., owned a construction company and always had one. As a child, riding around town in the bed of the truck felt like a free carnival ride, the wind whipping past the smiling faces of my siblings and me. The delight of waving smugly at the losers walking to their destinations. Then, the laws changed and forced us into the overcrowded safety of the interior cabin. Inside, where there was no more joy.

***

One late afternoon in the early fall of my 10th-grade year, my older brother Tony Jr. and I were taking a routine nap on our respective mauve couches in the living room. Our daily recovery routine was from the frigid, early morning excursions to the bus stop each day. After an hour or two, I'd get up to do my homework and chores while Tony watched TV.

We awoke groggily to familiar honking and vibrations from the driveway, signaling an unusual midweek visit from our father. Tony sent me out to investigate. I climbed into the passenger side of my dad's red pickup truck to see what he wanted. Dad was dressed in his work clothes and smelled of fresh wood and builder's paint. Despite being the owner-operator of a construction company, Dad was always clean and usually overdressed. I'd once seen him take three showers in one Sunday. One to start the day, another after playing hoops with his friends, and a final one after his evening volleyball or tennis match. All that physical activity left him tall and slender when most men his age had Dad bods.

Inside his truck, Dad seemed agitated. That wasn't unusual. Dad was often irritable for seemingly little reason. Like me, he was a Taurus, stubborn. He dished out commands and expected you to comply.

"Go pack an overnight bag. Y'all are coming with me," Tony Sr. snapped.

I was concerned. We never stayed at Dad's house during the week, especially not on a school night. The visitation timing was for bimonthly weekends at best.

My parents' relationship had been marked by turbulence from their days as high school sweethearts. Confronted with an unexpected pregnancy at 19 and excommunicated from the Seventh-Day Adventist (SDA) church, they succumbed to societal and family pressures and wed only after establishing my brother's legitimacy. Dad was unfaithful, perhaps Mom too, and they'd get into fistfights while we three children hid behind a bathroom door. Their relationship had dissolved by the time I reached first grade.

Tony Sr. was a "Disney Dad" after that, with short outings and inconsistent weekend visits. He remarried when I was 13 and had my youngest sister when I was 18. My older siblings and I felt the effects of "second family syndrome" as complex emotional and interpersonal dynamics of old versus new lives went unaddressed and forced to merge.

Despite Dad's tall stature and brooding temperament, Mom was always the more immediate threat to us.

"Does Mom know we're leaving?"

Nothing was quite as distressing as finding myself entangled in the ongoing conflict between my parents. Their mutual animosity and equal allocation of blame toward the other for our circumstances created an emotionally challenging atmosphere. I wanted no parts.

"Yes!" Dad hissed with his brows in a thick furrow.

A part of me didn't believe him. Something must have happened to Mom. It was the only explanation.

"Is Mom okay?"

"Yes. *Your mother* is just fine," his voice hardened with sarcasm.

He'd drawn out the words with disdain that I could tell Mom had done something. It reminded me of another occasion when my father had appeared unexpectedly.

I was around 7 or 8 years old back then. That night, my mother had vanished without a trace, leaving our teenage babysitter, a white girl, and her concerned parents to wonder about her prolonged absence. I'm unsure who reached out to my father, and the details of that night remain a mystery. I remember that when my mother arrived home, Dad was furious, and our favorite babysitter disappeared forever.

Dad didn't like to be questioned, especially not by children. As the adult, he told you what he wanted. I had no answers as to why we were leaving with him. All I could do was comply and wait to get caught in the middle when the time came.

I returned to the house to relay the news to Tony. He asked the same questions I had and seemed equally dissatisfied with the answers.

We each packed our toiletries and a change of clothes into a small brown Kroger grocery bag and headed outside. I climbed into the middle beside Dad, and Tony Jr. sat by the door. Dad pulled out of the driveway but headed west instead of east, where his house was.

Where were we going?

That silent question was answered momentarily when we pulled into the alleyway beside Granny's gray-paneled house. Dad honked his horn, and we waited. The sun was setting, and a few moments later, Devon came outside carrying a full black garbage bag.

Tony and I elbowed each other slightly as she walked toward the passenger-side door.

Why does she have so much stuff?

Tony Jr. got out, tossed Dev's bag in the truck bed, and let her slide in next to me in the middle. The youngest, Tanya, was adopted and would have to stay with our grandparents. I locked eyes with Devon as she scooted next to me, but could only partially interpret the brief telepathic signal she sent.

"I know what happened," her eyes said.

That's all I got before Tony got back in on the end, and we drove off back through town. This time, we headed east.

We'd picked up McDonald's on the way to Dad's house in the countryside. We settled in at the kitchen island of the newly constructed hilltop home. My stepmother, Tamara, looked irritated as she fussed around the kitchen moving small appliances and wiping invisible crumbs from the spotless counters. We were supposed to hate our stepmom per Mom's coaching or perhaps the idea of her because I don't remember the two women meeting. I was disloyal to the campaign, seeing the good in Tamara as one of the few safe adults in my life. Like everyone else though, she didn't fully understand our circumstances and was more critical of the outward manifestations of our troubled home life with my siblings including future high school attrition and unplanned pregnancies.

Dad settled stiffly on a barstool at the end of his long kitchen counter, finally ready to fill us in on the day's events. We sat expectantly in a nervous row, waiting to hear the news. It was more like a headline.

"Your Mom got into some trouble. Y'all have to stay with me for a little while."

Whereas Mom tended to overshare the facts of life, Dad was old school. There was adult business and a child's place. Of course, I had a million questions, but Dad was intimidating when he was angry and I knew better than to ask. My mind ran its usual silent analytics.

This must be bad.

Where was Mom? Was she safe?

How long is "a while"? Why can't we stay at Granny and Pawpaw's?

Who would take care of our youngest sister, Tanya?

Where would we go after school? Dad lived too far away.

"How would we get more clothes?"

That last one I actually asked aloud. Tony Jr. and I had only packed one change of clothes, not knowing that we would never sleep another night in our childhood home again. Dad let out his frustration.

"Why didn't you bring more clothes?" he fumed.

"You said pack a bag," I replied softly.

Up to then, we'd never stayed more than a night or two at Dad's house. I had no reason to expect that time would be any different.

He dismissed us from the table, telling us to shower and get ready for bed, youngest to oldest.

After bathing, Dad chastised us for leaving a "mess." Confused, I peered into the bathroom. It was just as I'd left it with clear counters and towels hung. I thought I'd done a good job. Dad pointed to the small pools of water on the sink and floor near the tub, demanding we wipe it up. I didn't understand. Water would dry, that wasn't messy where we came from, a place to which we would never return thanks to that CPS visit and that was all right by me.

References

1. Briere, J., & Scott, C. (2015). *Principles of trauma therapy: A guide to symptoms, evaluation, and treatment* (2nd ed.). SAGE Publications.
2. Porter, S., & ten Brinke, L. (2008). Reading between the lies: Identifying concealed and falsified emotions in universal facial expressions. *Psychological Science, 19,* 508–514.
3. Vrij, A., Granhag, P. A., & Porter, S. (2010). Pitfalls and opportunities in nonverbal and verbal lie detection. *Psychological Science in the Public Interest, 11*(3), 89–121. https://doi.org/10.1177/1529100610390861

CHAPTER 5

Stop Acting Fresh

<u>Adverse Childhood Experience—Sexual Abuse</u>

Childhood sexual abuse as when an adult, relative, family friend, or stranger who is at least five years older than the child: touches or fondles the child's body in a sexual way, makes the child touch their body in a sexual way, attempts to have any type of sexual intercourse with the child.[1]

TATIANA WAS A 21-year-old, single, Black, Mexican biracial woman with twin 6-year-old daughters. She was a long-term patient that I worked with on and off for about two years for chronic depression. As an only child, she was raised by her mother and her stepfather, who had been in her life since she was a toddler. Both were an immense help to Tatiana in raising her children. She was also close with her biological father, who was remarried and had several younger children.

Tatiana carried a lot of shame about having been a teenage mother. As an adult, she had become a devout member of the conservative Church of Christ, which I'd conceptualized as an attempt to achieve her idea of redemption. However, despite her religious transformation, she still felt unworthy of love from healthy men. Instead, she was drawn back into an old, toxic, and abusive relationship with her child's father.

Tatiana was so conventionally beautiful that it was puzzling that she was clueless to this fact. My non-therapeutic voice wanted to ask her if she had ever *seen* herself. She got a lot of male attention but believed that it was because men saw her as "easy" since she already had children, so she avoided them. Her self-esteem was so low that she couldn't receive anything besides the put-downs her ex regularly gave her when she dropped off their daughters for visits. He'd eventually persuade her that no one else wanted her and convince her to sleep with him again.

(dis)Honor Thy Mother: Daughterhood, Dysfunction and Deliverance, First Edition. Bridgette Peteet.
© 2026 John Wiley & Sons, Inc. Published 2026 by John Wiley & Sons, Inc.

Tatiana would feel guilty and rush back to church three times a week, accompanied by some variation of fasting. This cycle would repeat every few months.

Tatiana had avoided discussing her childhood sexual abuse well into our time working together. She eventually shared that she was too ashamed to tell me her story aloud, so I gave her a little "homework." I asked her to journal her story and return it the following week. Writing seemed to have empowered her. When she returned with the tiny turquoise journal, I expected her to resist reading it and assign me the task. Instead, she shared that something in her had clicked. Writing down her story helped her realize it was not her fault. She read the story to me with a bravery that I'd always seen underneath it all.

An older female relative had molested Tatiana for four years when she was a child. It was sporadic and mainly occurred at large family gatherings where she could lure her away unnoticed. Her advances progressed to sexual assault when Tatiana was 11 years old. Her perpetrator convinced her that no one would believe her if she told. She never did. That is until she came to therapy.

Her sexual abuse left her feeling worthless, and she started seeking male attention early on. Tatiana began dating her child's father at the end of middle school and was pregnant with twins by the first year of high school. Tatiana's mother had accepted her daughter's news graciously. She helped Tatiana with childcare so she could finish high school and continued offering support and shelter thereafter. The mother–daughter duo was incredibly close. Tatiana told her mother everything, everything but this decade-old secret.

After sharing parts of her story with me and processing her experience, Tatiana wanted to take her healing even further. In her mind, to begin to let go of her trauma, she needed to tell her mother. Tatiana had seen that, so far, her abuser's words had not come true. Someone had believed her. I had. I provided psychoeducation about the connection between her abuse and early sexual activity. It was as if a huge burden had been lifted in telling her truth to me. Still, Tatiana feared her mother's reaction. She worried her mother might not respond positively to hearing such damning news about one of her relatives. She stressed that her mother would blame her, a common fear among childhood sexual abuse survivors.[2,3]

Like me, Tatiana knew that some mothers believe their daughters (or sons), but others don't. I know from personal experience, client reports, and research that caregivers often ask victim-blaming questions like, "What did you do to provoke him/her?" or say inappropriate things like, "You must have enjoyed it to let it go on so long." Some mothers minimize the abuse with statements such as, "It wasn't that bad" or "He didn't mean it because he was [drunk]." These responses may stem from their unresolved history of sexual abuse, denial, shame, fear of being alone, or economic dependence on the abuser. In the end, these kinds of responses deter survivors of sexual abuse from coming forward, and when they do, they are all too frequently retraumatized by a lack of belief and support.

On the surface, Tatiana's hesitation about telling her mother seemed entirely understandable. However, everything I'd been told about her convinced me she would find support. For a month, though, I helped Tatiana weigh the evidence. We role-played how she would reveal her secret. We rehearsed the best- and worst-case scenarios in her mother's response. I taught Tatiana how to prime her mother's response with a statement like, "I'm going to tell you something complicated, and I want you just to listen." In her own time, she was ready. She took a deep breath and marched out of my office, head high.

Tatiana returned to therapy the following week, slightly embarrassed. The revelation to her mother had felt anticlimactic. Tatiana had spent years building it up in her mind. As is typical with fear and anxiety, it far exceeded reality. Instead of disbelief, anger, or blame, her mother pulled Tatiana into a warm embrace. She cried with her daughter and inquired about her current well-being. It was a supportive, affirming, and nurturing response. Tatiana was blessed to have a healthy mother capable of doing this; however, fortune doesn't smile upon everyone similarly.

***

In the heart of my childhood home, the living room buzzed with energy as a gathering of 6–8 adult relatives and neighbors encircled a small card table at its center. Amidst the laughter and chatter, my siblings and I, aged 5, 7, and 9, respectively, were reluctantly sent to bed. However, the allure of the festivities proved irresistible, and we hatched a plan to partake in the excitement without drawing the ire of the grown-ups.

Crafting a strategy akin to seasoned strategists, we orchestrated a rotation system, single, paired, and even triplicate formations that we would reshuffle with each successful mission downstairs. We abused the pretense of needing water, bathroom trips, or craving extra goodnight hugs and kisses. With each trip, we tested our luck, gauging the atmosphere and ensuring that our escapades remained undetected by our inebriated elders.

On my last trip through the living room, I gave my relatives one more kiss in my white printed onesie pajamas. I skipped one guest. He was a stranger. Adrian was caramel skinned with pea-green eyes and a short blondish afro. He was a little younger than my mother, in his mid-20s. I had never met a Black person with an eye color other than brown, and I'd never seen him before. I was intrigued.

My mother noticed my curiosity and avoidance and said, "Aw, Bridgette has her first crush."

At only seven years old, I wasn't sure what the word "crush" meant, but everyone's attention turned toward me, a gesture I hated decades later, even as I entered the sanctuary on my wedding day. Adrian and I both blushed at the declaration.

Nervously, I laughed off Mom's accusation and left to go to bed. Mom stopped me.

She teased, "Come back and give him a kiss."

My chuckle caught in my throat, but I assumed she was kidding. He wasn't a relative and wouldn't traditionally be included in that type of "goodnight." I reluctantly returned to the table and hugged Adrian quickly before dashing around the corner to the stairs. I had made it to the first platform when her subsequent demand hit my back. She had walked to the bottom of the steps, dragging a reluctant Adrian by the arm.

Sternly, she commanded, "Come down here and give him a kiss right now!"

Submissively, I returned to meet Adrian at the bottom of the stairs. Behind the wall, I was out of view of the other partygoers, no one to see my tears but him and my mother behind him, blocking his escape.

I stopped on the second step from the bottom, which left a disparity in height of about six inches. I mustered the courage to kiss him on the cheek and attempted to bolt back up the stairs a third time. This time, I did not make it as far.

Mom now commanded, "Give him a *real* kiss!"

Blinded with tears and frozen with fear, I hoped my reaction would sober her. It did not.

"Right NOW!" my mother persisted.

I slowly and reluctantly closed the distance between him and me. He looked embarrassed but licked his lips in preparation, a gesture I loathed from that day forward, though green eyes continued to fascinate me. My mouth met his moist lips, and I recoiled while my feet stayed planted, waiting to see if the task had been satisfactory this time. My mother turned with a smile to confirm to her guests that the deed was done. Around the corner, the room erupted in a howl, breaking my daze.

I took off as fast as I could, trying not to slip on the plastic bottoms on the feet of my pajamas. I flew past my siblings and ignored their inquiries, making it safely underneath the covers of my twin bed. Devon was across from me, and Tony was camping on the floor. They asked what had happened again, but I shook my head in the darkness. They likely assumed that I had finally been the one to get into trouble for going downstairs one too many times. In some ways, they would've been right. I cried until my sobs became hiccups, and a smile came across my innocent face.

"Did this count as my first kiss?" I wondered.

This type of confusion about intimacy would remain consistent throughout my childhood.

***

In the 5th grade, the girls and boys were separated to watch a movie about physical development starring the actress who had played "Annie." By then, Annie looked nothing like the redheaded child in the movies, whose life as an orphan reminded me of mine and gave me false hope that someone rich might adopt me one day. (The sun will come out tomorrow? Will it, though? Maybe next year.)

After sharing what I'd learned at school that day, Mom strode over to the tall bookshelves in the front room of our house and retrieved a giant textbook from her time training as a medical assistant. She flipped to the middle section, revealing page after page images of sexually transmitted infections on adult genitalia.

"This is herpes," Mom pointed out.

My eyes widened. I'd never even seen a penis, let alone one covered in clusters of overlapping lesions. It was a shock to my 10-year-old brain. For a long time after that, I assumed all of them looked deformed and diseased. It became an accidental abstinence advertisement. It also made me suspicious of asking my mother any other questions about human development or sex for fear of her extreme response.

On a long car ride one afternoon, my aunt read everyone's horoscope from the back of a women's magazine. Both my mom and aunt are Aries. My aunt turned to me and asked me my sign. I didn't know what that meant, so I shrugged. She scanned the page, looking for the one that captured my birthdate. I was a Taurus.

The predictions centered on relationships, love, and luck. I don't recall anything memorable from Mom or April's readings, but I remember part of mine.

"….enjoys oral sex," my aunt, five years my senior, turned to me with wide humor-filled eyes.

They burst into a cackle. I chuckled uncomfortably at the mention of "sex" but had no idea what the combination meant.

"What does that mean?" I asked awkwardly.

April repeated the phrase as if I hadn't heard her. I stared at her blankly.

"What does oral mean?" Mom tried to help.

"Mouth," I replied.

"And you know what sex is," Mom said definitively.

In theory, yes, I knew what parts were involved, but at 12, I was too young to know about the mechanics of it all.

"So, put that together," she concluded.

"Mouth sex?" I offered the answer with no improved understanding.

"STOP PLAYING STUPID BRIDGETTE!" Mom yelled, startling me.

I left it alone. I wasn't faking. I didn't understand.

Mom's response was probably related to her underlying discomfort. Mom presented as liberal and rampant, but underneath, she'd been socialized through her parents and the church that sex was a taboo topic. Her extremeness represented a defiance of her upbringing, but her anger revealed her uneasiness. Whatever the case, she silenced me, pushing me further into an internal world that kept me from asking any other questions about my body, love, or sex at a time when I was rapidly developing.

I didn't tell Mom for three months when I got my period in the 9th grade.

She had never heard about my first kiss on the campgrounds of our church conference that same summer.

She never met my first "real" boyfriend in college.

Meanwhile, Mom tried to make the extreme seem normal. I was in middle school when Mom got a strategically placed tattoo honoring her third husband, Ricky. She couldn't reach it. She assigned Devon or me the unappealing task of smearing a Vaseline-covered tongue depressor over her wound and covering it with plastic cling wrap.

Even in play, her touch was never restorative. Mom would say that I was "sensitive" when tears formed after she pinched and twisted the skin on my inner arms or legs. She'd bite us on our butts, hard enough to leave teeth marks in what was supposed to be play. She forced us to kiss her on the lips into adulthood. I hated it. My stomach would turn, a natural aversion that I more safely attributed to germaphobia in the concealment of my true feelings.

Devon was still in high school when our mother bought us gold lamé bikini underwear for Christmas. We held the panties up by the strings, eyes bulging toward each other in a silent sisterly message of distaste.

"Were we strippers?" our eyes asked.

Annoyed by our lack of gratitude, Mom quipped, "You all are just uptight!"

Careful not to further trigger her with any more negative feedback, we opened our matching stiletto combat boots with much more performative enthusiasm. However, I couldn't fake the same level of eagerness when she took me to an adult entertainment store that year.

Seeing the sign as we pulled into the strip mall parking lot, I hung my head and pleaded, "Mom, no."

She brushed me off, saying, "Bridgette, you're too prissy."

I wanted to stay in the car, but she denied my request.

After stuffing my mother into a black corset, I forcibly drew the line at her request to try out the ceiling-mounted harness displayed in the middle of the store. Shaking the prospective image out of my head and saying, "No…No…NO!" I steered Mom away by the back of the arm and was relieved that she allowed me to coax her out of the store.

***

I stayed at my mother's house in Columbus one fall weekend in high school. We were all looking forward to a visit with my great, great Aunt Vi. My grandparents were bringing the 100-plus-year-old woman by on an outing from the nursing home. Hungry, I came bouncing down the stairs to the kitchen before anyone arrived. I was 15 and growing curves where flatness had once resided for far too long in my teenage mind. After saving to get my hair done and wearing a semi-fashionable outfit that day, I felt more confident than usual.

I met his slimy eyes as I turned the corner at the bottom of the stairs. Ricky startled me since he had been standing out of my line of sight like a toddler with a distended abdomen. He was unfazed by my fright. He was staring at me, saying no words and revealing his rotted front tooth in a smirk. I instantly felt uncomfortable in my burgundy, plaid body suit and jeans and had left the denim shirt over it unbuttoned. I looked for an escape. There was none. I looked for help. There was no one.

As a young teen, I'd repeatedly fought off one cousin after three years of groping. Only my threat to tell finally stopped him. But, I was out of my depth with an adult man, my mother's husband no less. I'd heard that predators prey on the weak, so I pretended to be strong.

I asked him, "WHAT?" with all the Black girl sass and neck rolling I could muster.

My shakiness was giving me away, though. Ricky remained silent as he continued to scan my body up and down. I gulped and continued my charade, but he saw right through my bravado.

Fear of being found out had immobilized my previous abuser, and it seemed to be my only remaining weapon. I declared, "I will tell!"

This slowed his fixation, and I ran past him into the living room. I'd physically escaped but felt mentally trapped. With newfound clarity, my sisters' strange behavior came rushing back to my mind.

While visiting my mother's house, I shared a room with Devon, sleeping beside her unframed mattress on the low-pile carpeted floor. Devon seemed so relieved when I visited, but her nighttime rituals had changed in the short time we'd lived apart. She was frazzled and stressed at night. She'd turn off the light, nearly jump from the switch to her mattress, and tuck herself tightly under the covers in one fell swoop. We used to sleep in silence to hear anything coming in the night, but now she preferred noise from the radio above her head. Noise to drown out her fear, but fear of what? Her anxieties transferred to me, and I covered my head in anticipation of some unknown peril. Perhaps this was life in the capital city of Columbus and the best way to cope with outside dangers; only the danger lived inside the house.

***

My mother started to operate some informal boarding house for stray kids she met at the health clinic where she worked when I was in the 4th grade. She'd trade cash for food stamps with their parents and offer to take in their children for a weekend and eventually one kid for half a year. We didn't understand and wanted to know why, but in those days, you could not ask these questions of your parents. You gave up your bed for the distressed pregnant teenager with beautiful dark skin and long braided hair. You accepted the angry older boy Owen as your "brother" because your mother said.

Owen, 12, was in the 5th grade with my 11-year-old brother Tony. I was nine years old and a grade behind them. Owen was tall, dark-skinned, and wore the beginnings of a "tail" at the base of his faded hairstyle. His academic difficulties were immediately apparent. He could hardly read and struggled with math. We agreed with my mother's assessment that the city public schools he'd come from had failed him. But he was also angry. He once bloodied his knuckles, punching the wired, reinforced glass of our elementary school courtyard window because he was aggravated with his teacher. With my early helping skills, I suggested that he should punch something softer next time. That way, there'd be no pain or property damage, and he wouldn't get into trouble. I had far oversimplified Owen's issues.

One morning, just before school, I was curling my short, frizzy bangs two rooms away when I heard a loud thud. Startled, I quickly came around the corner and saw bright red blood squirting from my baby kitten's white neck as it seized on the yellow linoleum floor. Owen was standing over the flailing kitten, watching. I screamed hysterically for my mother to come downstairs and help. Everything was running in slow motion. Owen said he had climbed on a chair to get something from the top of the freezer. He'd "accidentally" landed on the kitten when he jumped down.

He had nothing in his hands. He retold the story with no emotion. Mom and Tony put the kitten in a box and rushed to the vet, where they couldn't revive her. I was distraught. We spent the day at Granny's house, skipping a school day.

On a walk across town one fall day, some other children and I shared our "Crazy Owen" stories. We welcomed the break when he would go home to visit his family in the city. We all agreed that he was bad news. As we vented, I let a story slip.

One day, I'd walked into Devon's bedroom and saw two tangled feet behind the closet wall. Owen's feet were pointing down, and Devon's feet were pointing up. I'd been forced into that position before and knew what it meant.

I'd yelled, "GET OFF OF HER!"

He startled, sitting up from behind the wall, making some excuse for the scene I could not hear in my rage. I followed my sister and never let him be alone with her again. Naïvely, I thought I had fixed the problem.

Two days after my walking confession, Mom and her 2nd husband William called a family meeting, beckoning each child into the front room for an interrogation; Owen first, then Devon, Tony, and me. I whispered to Tony when he returned and sat beside me, asking him what was wrong. He shook his head and wouldn't give me any clues. Since Owen was first, I figured it was something he had done again. Then, it was my turn in the chair.

I slowly entered the living room and sat across from Mom and William. Mom relayed the story I had told the others days before. My heart sank.

They began to grill me about what I had seen.

"Have you seen him do this other times? Why didn't you tell us? Why didn't you protect your baby sister?"

In my young mind, I believed I had come up with a reasonable solution to protect my sister *and* not get my new "brother" into trouble. That's what we did in our family: keep secrets. Wasn't it?

Mom continued, laying the guilt on thick.

"You are the oldest."

I wasn't.

"You're her big sister. It is your job to take care of her."

Caregiving was actually Mom's job.

I felt defensive. My mother was the one who'd brought a troubled child to live with us. Seeing what I saw wasn't my responsibility. I wanted to tell Mom it was her fault, but I knew better. Problems were never her fault. Ever.

Devon, Owen, and I got whipped with the extension cord that day. Devon was given a few licks for "letting him do it." She was five years younger than Owen but held equally guilty. I got two swats for not telling. My mother seemed to whip Owen as if to say, "You are in trouble, but you're also not my child." She didn't lose it on him like she'd done with us when the crimes were this high.

Owen wasn't sent back home to his family. Sometimes, we were allowed to go home with him. We were exposed to a lot on those visits, things that seemed odd then but would become normal to us in a few years. He lived with us until, one day, his mom wanted him back. He left for the weekend. We never heard from or saw our "brother" again.

Owen likely had an oppositional defiant disorder, a childhood behavioral disorder characterized by a consistent pattern of angry, irritable, and defiant behavior, often directed toward parents, teachers, or other authority figures.[4] These behaviors go beyond the normal boundaries of childhood disobedience and can significantly affect a child's social, academic, and family life. The exact causes of oppositional defiant disorder are not fully understood, but it's believed to be influenced by a combination of genetic, environmental, and neurological factors.[5–7] Our chaotic home environment would have done little to quell his challenges.

***

After Ricky's stares that day, I started watching my sisters more closely. Devon, at 13, seemed the same in the light of day; she presented a brave front on the city streets as I skittishly jumped at men catcalling to us. Tanya was only three then, but I watched her, too. Everything she did became suspicious. She'd sit splayed about in her nightgown and resisted when we told her to sit "ladylike." Was that a sign that something had happened to her? I kept watching both of my little sisters for more apparent signs. What signs, I had a few ideas, but speculation was insufficient.

A few months later, when Devon visited me at Granny's house one weekend, I immediately noticed a bruise on her cheek. I asked her what happened, thinking she had been in a fight at her new school.

Numbly, she responded with one word, "Ricky."

Her brief response set a bomb off inside me. I felt angry, sick, scared, and guilty that my fears were true. I wanted him to die, but more so, I wanted to kill him. I'd hold onto that wish for almost the rest of my life.

Devon began to relay the story that she'd told Mom. They were riding in the car, and Mom had noticed the bruise much like I did. However, instead of the numb response Devon had given me, she broke down sobbing into her hands and named her abuser.

"Ricky!" Devon burst in a moment of relief. Her secret was out. Mom would save her now. But Debra jumped to Ricky's defense before Devon could say another word about her abuse.

Debra quipped, "Shut the f@*# up! He was just playing with you; stop being so dramatic!"

Hearing this story, my anger shifted from Ricky to Debra like a tsunami. Silently, she was Debra now. She was no longer my mother.

How could a 'mother'....?, I thought.

Why would a 'mother'....? I stopped.

Because Debra was not a mother. She was a woman who had kids.

Mom was 36 with four dependents but living for herself and herself only. Everything I'd suspected about her was solidified in that moment. Something was wrong with her. It was the second major shift in our relationship since I'd physically escaped her grasp less than a year prior. Her response to Devon made me unravel. Debra did not even let her finish the story. She has *never* heard Devon's story. For that matter, neither have I.

I don't know if Devon wanted to tell, yet her silence was telling. She and I sometimes recounted our stories, most written off as lustful or incestuous abuse from male relatives close in age that did not seem to rise to the level of "trauma" in our minds. But her experience with Ricky was different. Ricky was an adult, a convicted pedophile, or so said the rumor. We'd visited him in prison while Mom was still married to and living with her second husband on what became semi-conjugal visits when she sent us to the restroom.

My mind constructs a story of Devon's abuse that I cannot bear to ask of her. It involves strategic victim selection, gaining access, building trust, and steady increases in physical touch that instills confusion but avoids sounding the alarm of danger. It has been so skillfully manipulated that by the time the assault comes, she thinks it was her fault, that she did something to entice him, that her mother won't believe her. Despite the evidence on her face, she would be right on that last count.

They say there is nothing more dangerous than a woman desperate for a man. Debra chose her man over her child. She continued her relationship with Ricky until some other issue eventually broke them up. In our house, there was no momentary reprieve or time to adjust and heal. It was onto the next relationship, the next predator just released from prison. This time, John got kicked away when he tried to touch Devon. He didn't last long; most men didn't. Thirteen of them in a 15-year span. The effects of Debra's love bombing only lasted so long. We'd enjoy the fruits of her short-lived mothering, a clean house, prepared meals, and fleeting moments of fun. We'd learned to brace ourselves from this parade of cohabitating males, to detach ourselves from any emotional investment in their presence. It wasn't personal; it simply cost us too much to care.

Some of my relatives found relief when Mom wedded a PK, preacher's kid, the same year I got married in 2003. Malik, her 4th husband, was mild-mannered with stable employment, which was undoubtedly a step up from the rest. Malik seemed to have a high emotional pain tolerance and purportedly didn't believe in divorce, though he'd already had one.

By then, I was off building my life and marriage at a safe distance from my family. Despite people singing Malik's praises and him doing nothing egregious, I was numb. He was no one to me. He was Mom's husband, not a "stepdad." I couldn't invest any part of myself in getting to know him. I was emotionally exhausted. It wasn't about him or his virtues. Debra was the common denominator; as usual, it was more of the same.

Debra was babysitting my toddler niece one night. She was tired, but my niece needed a bath. Malik was taking a shower, so Debra devised a seemingly simple solution. She placed the toddler girl into Malik's arms and told him to wash the baby simultaneously. He complied. Debra later relayed the tale of her ingenuity to Devon with pride.

Mom's joy faded when Devon immediately snapped, fully and wholly triggered. Debra was dumbfounded and defensive. Nothing had happened, and Malik was innocent. No one said he had. It wasn't the point. Mom didn't get it. She never would, but we saw the pattern of neglect and heedlessness. We couldn't unsee it or remain quiet about what was or could happen. Silence is a form of consent. We would not be complicit.

References

1. Centers for Disease Control (CDC). (n.d.). *Fast facts: Preventing adverse childhood experiences.* https://www.cdc.gov/violenceprevention/aces/fastfact.html

2. Rakovec-Felser, Z., & Vidovič, L. (2016). Maternal perceptions of and responses to child sexual abuse. *Slovenian Journal of Public Health, 55*(2), 124–130.

3. American Academy of Child & Adolescent Psychiatry. (n.d.). *Oppositional defiant disorder resource center: FAQ.* https://www.aacap.org/AACAP/Families_and_Youth/Resource_Centers/Oppositional_Defiant_Disorder_Resource_Center/FAQ.aspx

4. Zajac, K., Ralston, M. E., & Smith, D. W. (2015). Maternal support following childhood sexual abuse: Associations with children's adjustment post-disclosure and at 9-month follow-up. *Child Buse & Neglect, 44*, 66–75.

5. American Psychiatric Association. (2022). *Diagnostic and statistical manual of mental disorders* (5th ed., text rev.). https://doi.org/10.1176/appi.books.9780890425787

6. Cleveland Clinic. (n.d.). *Oppositional defiant disorder (ODD).* https://my.clevelandclinic.org/health/diseases/9905-oppositional-defiant-disorder

7. WebMD. (n.d.). *Oppositional defiant disorder (ODD).* https://www.webmd.com/mental-health/oppositional-defiant-disorder

CHAPTER 6

Look to Your Left and Your Right

Adverse Childhood Experiences and Environment

Our environment shapes the nature of our trauma. From family dynamics to community support, the social context in which we grow up plays a crucial role in either exacerbating or mitigating the effects of ACEs. Communities with deficient resources, inadequate housing, and community disruptions may worsen the effect of ACEs.[1-3]

I WALKED INTO the near-empty diner that night. There was something in the air. Something more than french fry grease. I followed my manager, Rob, to the back of the restaurant and through the kitchen to his tiny office. He was about 30, with prematurely balding spiky red hair and was built like the Tasmanian devil. Rob motioned me toward the pleather rolling chair and sat on the other side of the awkward wooden school desk.

When I woke up that morning, I had no idea I would be fired and fired on my day off, no less. I was a cliché. A year before, that catchphrase had appeared in the classic movie *Friday*, in which the rapper Ice Cube's character, Craig, got fired on his day off.

At 16, I had my first real job. I was a waitress. We were waitresses in those days, not servers. I'd started working when I was 12, babysitting my Uncle Joey's and then Uncle Brian's kids. In the years after and into college, I was a janitor, a housekeeper, a cashier, a receptionist, a telemarketer, and a home health aide. I worked because I needed to. I had shelter, living with my grandparents and later in the dorms, but I had to cover my basic needs. Clothes, shoes, transportation, toiletries, activities, and so forth made for a long list of needs on a child's limited budget.

As a waitress, I made $2.13 an hour plus tips. At about $5 an hour, it was close to minimum wage, yet not enough to move anyone out of poverty. The upside, cash tips. It was like getting paid instantly. We also got discounted food and ice cream sundaes that I took full advantage of. The downside was that I saw how the sausage was made. *Literally*. Kind of. Grease traps. Congealed ranch salad dressing. Sticky arms scooping ice cream. Tubs of wilted lettuce. The scary walk-in fridge that I was convinced housed a family of mice though I never saw them. I now understood why my Pawpaw had an aversion to dining out. The cherry on top of these questionable delectables was drama.

Who was stealing tables?
Whose turn it was to get a table?
Who was sleeping with whom?
Who was mean?
Who was lazy?

Lazy? It was me. I was lazy; at least, that's the rumor a new coworker started about me with the new manager. It was an unoriginal stereotype.

"Bridgette wipe the menus down," Rob barked on my first shift with him. He bragged about his come up from the fast food industry to a dine-in restaurant. Rob boasted about his ability to get older women, dating a 50-something-year-old waitress with the haggard appearance of a longtime smoker and sun-worshipper.

Before I could answer Rob, Kristy, the new waitress chimed in. "I'll do it." It was my second time working with Kristy. I'd helped train her on her first shift. She attended a rival county high school but seemed pleasant enough. I was grateful for the reciprocity. Since she was new, I had five tables, and she had two. I was sprinting around like crazy.

"No, Bridgette will do it," Rob barked through pursed lips.

I hurried to the front of the restaurant and wiped down a stack of menus sticky with faux maple syrup.

Less than an hour later, Rob came at me again, "Bridgette, refill the ice dispenser."

"I can do it for her," Kristy offered again before I could get an entire word out.

"NO! Bridgette WILL do it!" Rob snapped, not looking at me but letting me know his tone was for my ears.

I filled a tub with ice and climbed up the stepladder to load the top of the pop machine dispenser. Returning the empty ice tub to the kitchen, I passed my best friend Stacey. Friends since the start of high school, we had gotten jobs at the restaurant together.

"What's wrong with that guy?" I asked in a hushed tone.

Stacey's thin face turned pink. She hesitated.

"Before you got here today, Kristy told Rob that you were lazy."

My face felt as if it were changing colors. I had only worked with Kristy once before, when I'd shown her the ropes. She hardly had any tables that day, but I was "lazy." She'd reduced me to a stereotype and made it look true by volunteering for my assignments. Factually, though, she had time to offer because she wasn't doing anything.

I turned to storm through the swinging double doors of the kitchen, but Stacey stopped me with a reminder.

"She knows karate!" her brown eyes wide.

I paused a moment. I wasn't a fighter. Fights with my sister, Devon, didn't count, although she was known for body-slamming a boy during a childhood street fight so maybe it did. There was the time my 8th grade classmate Jeff punched me in the nose. I'd been yelling at him for throwing rocks at my little sister, Tanya, in the park. I'd sparred occasionally in karate classes in elementary school until a boy punched me in my developing chest. I lost all form and function of training and launched into the windmill fighting style before the teacher pulled me off of him. Then, there was Mom. Her go-to move had been to slap me across the face, leaving a red, hand-shaped mark each time. So, in my estimation, I could take a hit. But a fight? My mind said maybe. My pride didn't care. I never back down from bullies. Ever.

It slipped out before I could stop myself. Kristy had passed me for the third time, fake smiling on my face. I don't do phony exceptionally well. It's never been my strength.

Long before Will Smith's Academy Award infamous slap, I copied his words and told Kristy "Keep my name out of your mouth!"

I looked down into her eyes and held my stare. I was going for intimidation. Aggression is a common tool of the otherwise powerless.

Kristy's eyes widened, and she took one step back. It wasn't an offensive movement, as if preparing to strike. She'd shrunken away from me.

Huh, that fake-out worked.

Kristy left me alone after that, but Rob was just getting started.

While Rob let his girlfriend take multiple smoke breaks, he commanded me to clean underneath booth cushions, scrape gum from the underside of the tables, and scrub the bathroom toilets. His orders extended beyond the usual server chores. I dared question him once, and he yelled, "Because I said so!"

Rob wanted me to be afraid of him. I wasn't. I'd been through too much in my short time on earth. I felt empathy for Rob. He was at the height of his power, whereas I was just getting started. My dreams were much bigger than that diner.

***

"I want to go to Harvard and become a lawyer." This was my usual response when adults asked me what I wanted to be when I grew up. I was going to college. It was the one thing that no one doubted, not even my mother, or so it seemed. With all of that encouragement, there was still one problem. I didn't know *anything* about college.

Most of what I knew about Harvard came from its reputation and a highly offensive movie from 1986 called *Soul Man*. In the film, the white main character takes an overdose of tanning pills to steal a scholarship intended for a Black student.—Yes, Blackface. I didn't realize that it was offensive at the time, forgive my ignorance. I was more focused on Rae Dawn Chong's portrayal of "Sarah," a severe and studious Black woman working hard to make it to school. I wanted to be her, minus the baby (another cringy stereotype in the movie). "Sarah" made Harvard feel reachable. Never mind that I had no idea how to get into the university down the street, let alone an Ivy League institution 11 hours away from rural Ohio.

At about the same time, *The Cosby Show* aired. Phylicia Rashad, as Clare Huxtable, modeled a successful Black woman in her roles as a lawyer, wife of a doctor, and mother. She was my end goal. I'm often told I resemble her. Then, the spinoff, A Different World, showed a step in between. The series depicted students' personal lives at a fictitious historically Black college (though I'm embarrassed to admit that I thought Hillman College was a real school for way too long). A school friend and I would play "college," mimicking what we saw on the screen. We'd sit in her bedroom and pretend to study using a giant dictionary for our textbook. But then, my friend went too far and asked me to play her college boyfriend. *Welp, time to go.*

Still, my imagination put me there. In college. On the campus. In the dorm. In the classroom.

Being a lawyer was my default career. It, along with doctor, was the main "successful" career options that I knew about. The certainty that I had no desire to handle bodily fluids made the decision easy. Doctor was out, well physician anyway.

My family shared my law school dreams but had no idea what I needed to do to get there. Like when Granny, ever helpful, videotaped the entire O.J. Simpson murder trial for me so I could use it for school one day. Granny had all of the "trial of the century" recordings stacked neatly inside a banker's box, preparing for my future. In the meantime, I'd heard through peers in my honors English class that I should talk to my high school guidance counselor about college.

I was nervous when I sat down across from the older man. I thought guidance counselors were for kids who'd gotten into trouble. They'd checked in on me once after child protective services (CPS) removed us from our childhood home the year before.

"How are you?"

"Fine."

"Great." Moving on.

I didn't know their other job was to help you get into college.

The guidance counselor stretched his long legs over the top of his desk and leaned back in his chair. I'd asked him how to apply to college. He stared toward the ceiling, telling me stories about his son at Brown and the other at Purdue, not the chicken company of the same name with a different spelling. After 10 minutes, our time was up. All I had learned was that getting into the Ivy League was "hard." He'd been talking about top tier schools. My question was about *any* school. I didn't know how to apply.

As if magic, after I took the PSAT, college brochures started arriving in the mail. I was thrilled as I collected the shiny, vibrant-colored pamphlets. It would be my only "tour" of most campuses. But, there it was on the last pages—how to apply.

As my oversized manila envelope filled, a new question replaced the first. There were hundreds of colleges in Ohio and thousands around the country. How was I supposed to decide where to go?

I'd brought over the stack of brochures to check out with my cheery but frank stepmom. Tamara was the closest person in my life who had a college degree. She also had a perpetual smile, sharp humor, and a penchant for gentle judgment.

"Capital University looks nice in the pictures. Where's that at?" I'd scanned the brochure cover to cover and couldn't find the location.

"You don't know where that is?" Tamara questioned with a raised eyebrow. "It's in the capital. Columbus," she said as if it were obvious. Heat rose to my face. Of course, I knew the capital of my home state. I just hadn't put two and two together. I felt stupid. From then on, I played it safe—comments, not questions. Tamara helped me weigh and weed my college options down to a comfortable few.

Other than a limited regional college tour with a group from high school, I visited one other school with my friend Elizabeth and her family. We fell in love with the sprawling green hills of the yard at a nearby public institution and applied.

Back in my hometown, I was starting to feel caught between two worlds, unprepared for the one and pulling away from the other.

In my senior year of high school, after basketball cheerleading ended, I got a job at a local dry cleaner. Less than three months ago, I was there when my boss Mike announced that he had some exciting news.

"Congratulations, we're promoting you to manager," he announced excitedly. Mike was dressed in a button-down dress shirt and khakis like he was going to the corporate office instead of bagging soiled suits at the dry cleaner's drop-off. He had been promoted to district manager at Swan Cleaners. Mike was 40. I'd just turned 18.

Mike covered the morning shift, and I worked after school from 3 to 7 p.m. It was an easy job. We collected dirty clothes and returned the clean ones. We didn't do any on-site washing except for occasional bulk laundry from long-term guests across the parking lot at the hotel.

"You scored a perfect ten on the test for your job application a few months ago. No one gets a perfect. The folks at the district office were impressed," Mike said, flashing his bright teeth.

That disclosure surprised me. The one-page test consisted of math word problems about how much change to give back to a customer and a question matching letter and number combinations correctly. It was 4th-grade level math at best.

"Now that you're about to graduate, you can take over this location," Mike beamed, rocking back on his heels.

We stood eye to eye as I tried to figure out what missteps Mike must have made in life. He was a polished and polite white man and had been the manager for four years. He had a wife and two children. I didn't understand how I was fit to be his successor. I was flattered. I'd come a long way from that first job as a waitress two years earlier, where I was definitely not a candidate for promotion.

Thinking back to that final day with Rob at Friendly's, I remember him calling my Grandparent's house one Saturday evening in the late summer before my junior year. He wanted me to come in right away. I couldn't. It was the Sabbath, and not working on Saturdays was a condition of living at my Grandparent's house. They only let me do cheerleading because I had been doing it long before I moved in with them.

Rob called back again two hours later. This time, he was less successful in concealing his anger and demanded to know why I wasn't there yet. Resenting the intrusion and ready to defend, Pawpaw and my aunt, April, drove me around the corner to the restaurant after sunset.

Once situated behind the desk in the cramped manager's office, Rob slammed the printed paper in front of me. He jabbed his swollen pointer finger toward a teeny box in the middle of the page. It was a newspaper from a nearby town. The opening sentence in the area he had pointed out read,

"Friendly's should change its name to Unfriendly."

I finished the short paragraph. In brief, it said that two waitresses had been rude, and the patron had "tipped accordingly."

My stomach sank. The customer had heard me. "This guy is all up in our conversation," I'd told another waitress a month earlier.

"What do you know about this?" Rob demanded.

"I'm not sure. Are you asking everyone?" I offered, not knowing what evidence the prosecution had.

"I called the customer, and he said it was you."

"He said my name?" I doubted it.

"Well, no," Rob stammered, his red face now matching the thin fuzz atop his head.

"He said it was a white girl and a 'Black girl'!" He whispered "Black" as his face ran through the colors of the rainbow.

"The customer said that *I* said that."

"Uh, no. He said one of you."

"OK, so who's the other person?"

"I don't know," Rob stuttered.

"I don't remember being rude to one of my customers."

"He said you were on a break."

"Was I on a break or serving his table?" Rob knew it would be unusual for me to be on a break if I had a table of eight.

"I don't know!" He snapped.

"Who was I talking to? Does anyone else remember this?"

"I didn't ask anyone else yet." Rob quipped, clearly not pleased with my inquiries.

"Interesting. Could it have been the other person who said it?"

"Yes, it's possible!" Rob agreed, fully crimson now. "I'll have to investigate more. You're suspended until then." He rushed through the last part as if he'd been waiting to say it. He'd wanted to say it since he first met "lazy" me. My questions had thrown off his plans, but his closing declaration reset the power imbalance.

I walked out through the restaurant, holding back my tears. Rob lumbered behind as if he was throwing me out.

I got back in the van and let go. Through my sobs, I told Pawpaw and April what happened. April jumped out before Pawpaw, or I could stop her. She claimed that she was going to get ice cream. We knew better.

I have no idea what April said to Rob when she went inside. I could see him through the window, shifting from leg to leg and holding his hands open and out as if he now didn't want the problem he'd created.

Two years later, at the dry cleaner, I could see who Rob had been more clearly. He was a financially stressed-out adult with few choices in life who had taken out his frustrations on me. Mike was a better boss than Rob but similar in that he also underestimated me. I realized even more that a career in customer service wasn't the future I wanted. I had to go to college. I was going to college. I had gotten in.

I let Mike finish his grand manager promotion speech.

"Thank you for your offer. I'm flattered, but I also have some good news. I was just accepted into an early college program. I leave in two weeks."

The smile faded from Mike's face. "Oh. Congratulations. I'm surprised to hear that."

"Really? I've been telling you I was going to college all this time. At best, I would've been leaving this fall."

"Um, I don't know. I thought maybe your plans had changed," he stammered.

My plans *had* changed, for the better. I was leaving town early.

***

We pulled the navy blue, oversized conversion van into the loading dock of my new dorm. Pawpaw, Granny, and Dev hobbled out after the long trip. My new dorm, Two Towers, perfectly named, cast an intimidating shadow over my head.

I'd moved a two-hour drive or a four-hour Greyhound bus ride from home. Close enough that I could get back in an emergency and far enough that no one would visit me without calling first.

A tall, dark-skinned boy rolled an industrial-sized canvas laundry cart toward the back of the van. The boy was one of the peer mentors for the summer bridge program. His eyes widened behind his goggles when Pawpaw opened the double doors.

"There's no way all of this is going to fit."

My ears burned as if I'd already messed up on my first college exam. *Impostor* rang in my head. I'd packed all my worldly possessions in the back row and rear of the van. It was a miracle it all hadn't tumbled out onto the ground of the loading dock. I'd cleared out my entire bedroom. Dev had moved into my old room at Granny and Pawpaw's, finally away from Mom. I felt like I had a one-way ticket out of town, and there was no going back.

The boy suggested that we look at the room first. Six floors later, we arrived in front of a beige metal door. My name hung above it, and a brightly colored "Welcome." I unlocked the door with one of the two keys the front desk staff gave me. The other was for the entrance to the building. Using a little too much force, the door swung open 90° before clanging against the metal twin XL bed behind it.

The room length extended three feet past the foot of the bed, with enough space for a study desk and chair. A built-in closet dresser combo was on my right. The room aesthetics gave off prison vibes. But I smiled. I was free, no longer a prisoner. Everything fit perfectly.

I spent eight weeks on campus that summer with 30 Black kids from varying cities around the state. We took classes, learned strategies for academic success, and participated in cultural events, including a Rites of Passage ceremony. Ultimately, I'd earned seven credit hours and a 4.0 GPA. College felt easy.

By the time fall first-year orientation came around, it felt redundant. I knew my way around most of the 953-acre campus. I'd made one or two close friends and 50 more acquaintances. That summer, almost all students on campus were Black, either program participants, peer mentors, or athletes. We'd bonded in the heat and humidity of June and July in northeast Ohio. Then August came, and it snowed.

That's what the older students called it when our little cultural bubble burst, and the campus flooded with white students. The atmosphere flipped in a single weekend, move-in days.

Some of my friends had gone to all-Black high schools and were shocked to find themselves now in a predominately white environment. I was used to it. It was what I'd come from.

When we walked down Main St., a pickup truck drove past with its occupants yelling, "Go home, Ni**ers!" I rolled my eyes and kept strolling. One friend strained to devise an alternative slur that she must've heard while the other friend melted into a seat on the curb, face in hands.

My friends and I looked like chocolate sprinkles on a vanilla sundae in the main auditorium for orientation that day. It would be a day-long introduction to college life with tours, scheduling information, and presentations. We had done that already, so I half-listened until something caught my ear.

"Look to your left and your right. Two of you won't be here at graduation," some administrator remarked from the stage down below.

The eyes of the pale faces on both sides of me widened. A few new brown faces looked scared, too. I had been in their shoes two months prior. I was worried for them, not me. I was confident that I could do college. Too confident.

***

That moment in the auditorium came back to me 20 years later. I situated my coffee, laptop, and supply tote on the front conference tables as participants trailed into the room for the day-long diversity training. I began, as always, with the requisite introductions: name, position, background, and one interesting fact. We'd made our way almost around the room when my eyes met familiar ones. Her nametag said, "Chantel." I smiled as she introduced herself.

"I'm Chantel Jacobs, and I'm a support services specialist. I've been with the county for three months. One interesting fact about me is that I'm a great cook."

"And you went to college with me, right?" I asked, perched on the edge of a long table.

Chantel drew her head back. "How do you remember that?"

"I have no idea," I shrugged.

"I only went there for one semester. I got homesick, and my mom let me stay home after the winter break," she shared.

Eager to catch up, I approached Chantel at lunch. She told me that she regretted listening to her mother. She hadn't known that homesickness was normal and would lessen with time. Chantel never returned to school to finish her degree but had been employed full-time since.

"Now look at us," she noted. "You went all the way in school, and I never left home again."

I didn't know what to say—the nostalgic moment had turned awkward.

"Well, it's never too late to return to school." I silver-lined her regrets and retreated to my facilitator's corner with a tinge of survivor guilt or remorse for having escaped my childhood circumstances.[4]

References

1. Danielson, R., & Saxena, D. (2019). Connecting adverse childhood experiences and community health to promote health equity. *Social and Personality Psychology Compass, 13*(7), e12486. https://doi.org/10.1111/spc3.12486
2. Ellis, W. R., & Dietz, W. H. (2017). A new framework for addressing adverse childhood and community experiences: The building community resilience model. *Academic Pediatrics, 17*(7), S86–S93. https://doi.org/10.1016/j.acap.2016.12.01

3. Pinderhughes, H., & Davis, R. (2018). From adverse childhood experiences to adverse community experiences: Addressing and preventing community trauma. In J. D. Osofsky & B. M. Groves (Eds.), *Violence and trauma in the lives of children: Prevention and intervention* (pp. 215–234). Praeger/ABC-CLIO.

4. American Psychological Association (APA) (2018). *Survivor guilt*. APA Dictionary of Psychology. https://dictionary.apa.org/survivor-guilt

CHAPTER 7

Lessons Learned

Adverse Childhood Experiences and Adult Relationships

The effects of ACEs extend into adulthood, influencing how we form and navigate intimate partner relationships. Childhood trauma can shape our emotional responses, attachment styles, and patterns of trust, often creating challenges in building healthy, supportive partnerships.[1]

PICKING A COLLEGE major seemed easy enough based on no knowledge of careers: prelaw. Only there was no pre-law major at my university. I had to pick something else. Undecided, I felt too risky as if I didn't know what I wanted to do. I'd never heard of political science, and when I did, the name sounded boring. I had zero interest in politics. I eventually landed on criminal justice.

I was excited when I got to my criminal law class in junior year. The course description aligned with everything I'd seen on TV about lawyers. This was it. My chance. I had to do well.

I routinely formed study groups or found a study buddy in most of my classes to help me stay on track. In this night class, most were older, nontraditional students with full-time jobs. I'd learned that finding time to study with them was tough.

Rajiv sat next to me, the only other young, brown person in the class. Based on stereotypes, I assumed that he was intelligent. He had a unique minty smell and seemed obsessed with drinking Pepsi. I invited him to set up a study group with me after class.

As we exited the building, a gust of icy January wind hit us like a wall. I bid my farewell to my new friend and turned toward the walking path leading to my dorm on the far side of the campus.

As I was about to head off into the shadows, Rajiv's voice called out, breaking the silence. He offered to give me a ride back to my dorm, and, for a moment, I hesitated. The path ahead looked ominous, dark corners and eerie silence, and he was a stranger. I weighed my options. I glanced at Rajiv, considering my decision. He was slightly smaller than me, and I had about 20 lb on him. That thought gave me a slight sense of reassurance. If things took an unexpected turn, I believed I could handle myself.

Rajiv was a perfect gentleman that night. We got into a groove over the next two months. Class, study, get a ride home. As I got to know him, it turned out that Rajiv wasn't addicted to Pepsi after all. His addiction was much worse. He was obsessed with chewing tobacco. That explained his persistent minty odor. He used the pop cans to catch his spit. He kept a can on the floor during class and study sessions. I'd stare at the can as it transformed in my mind into a 55-gallon metal drum of saliva with wet brown bits rolling down the side. I'd talk myself down by focusing on the big picture. The midterm. It would be half of our grade.

Our professor strolled through the six aisles right after Spring Break, calling names and passing back our midterm exams. In between, he announced that there would only be a tiny curve. I sighed in frustration. Some *nerd* had scored a 97% and messed it up for everybody. My grade now rested too heavily on the final. Scores typically fall during finals as too many things compete for space in your memory. I'd have to work twice as hard.

Rajiv got his test back first. He turned his paper toward me—a 74%. I raised an eyebrow. He looked calm. My stomach sank. We'd worked harder than a C. It should at least be a B. The test hadn't felt difficult.

The towering professor reached my desk a minute later. He looked down at me. He looked back at the paper. He looked at me again.

"Bridgette?"

"Yes."

The professor's eyes widened.

Ughhhhh, I must've failed. Tears were at the ready in the corner of my eyes.

"Good job," he quipped, laying the exam face on my half desk.

The professor hadn't said anything directly to anyone else when handing back the exams. His comment caused several heads to turn in my direction.

I dragged the paper across the desk toward my chest. A large, red circle with the number 97% filled the top right corner of the page. I felt the blood drain from my face before quickly flipping the test back over.

"What is it?" Rajiv whispered with concern in his eyes.

I flashed the corner of the page in his direction and stuffed it into my book bag so no one else could see.

"Good job! I knew it was you. You're so smart," he smiled a congratulations with brown specks gathering at his gum line. I was happy that he was proud of me and not jealous. It was refreshing. I'd broken up with a boy in high school after sharing that I'd earned straight As and he'd accused me of calling him "stupid" in the next breath. I was quick to cut guys off. I *was* going to need a new study partner though. Rajiv was dragging down the team.

As we hurried through the cold night to Rajiv's car after class, I asked him what happened with his exam. We'd studied together, and he should've done better. Rajiv shared that he had been distracted. My shoulders sank. I felt like a careless friend. I had no idea he was going through something. I apologized for missing his struggle. He scraped the car windows, and I sat inside, shivering in the northeastern air. My mind started ticking through ways to help him ace the final. My savior complex was strong in those days, a compulsion to save others.[2]

The car was finally starting to warm up when he got back inside; only he didn't put it into gear. I looked over to see what he was doing. His upper body was turned in my direction, and he stared at me through the darkness.

"There's something I've been wanting to do."

He grabbed the back of my head and lunged toward me, all while trying to pull me in for a kiss. I used my free left to stiff arm him and halt his forward movement. I wriggled my head away from his embrace, grateful he didn't resist my escape.

"Why did you do that?" I spit as I gathered my belongings and made a hasty retreat into the winter night.

I didn't tell anyone what had happened. A part of me felt like I'd brought it on myself, and I rationalized that it could've been worse. Still, I felt a flicker of pride. I had stood up to him instead of giving in to the unwanted advances of a man just to avoid his wrath or simply disappointment. That moment marked a shift in me. I was beginning to confront the people-pleasing tendencies that had long governed my life.

Those tendencies weren't random—they were survival mechanisms shaped by a childhood where safety always felt fragile and conditional. My needs had been secondary to the unspoken rules of staying small and avoiding disruption. But those rules no longer served me. I was starting to break free.

***

At the end of Spring of my senior year of college, I walked into my Policing final. Strangely, three guys I knew from a Black Greek organization were waving frantically in my direction from the back of the classroom. What were they doing there? They must be lingering from the previous class, I thought.

I'd dated one of them on a rebound from my first college boyfriend, Jason, and felt obligated to be polite. So, I smiled and waved back, slowly realizing they were gesturing for me to come and sit with them. They were there for the final. We'd just finished four months of biweekly classes, and these guys hadn't been to one. This must be their Hail Mary attempt to make up for it.

"Bridgette. Come sit with us," the rebound boy beckoned loudly, and the rest of their plan became apparent.

Usually, slighting them would have felt like my social downfall. But getting expelled would not bear well for my future. A rapid calculation reminded me that I was finishing college in two days. I would never see them again.

I pretended not to hear their invitation and slid into a desk near the professor. Some other poor girl didn't process the scene fast enough and got caught in their web. I'd been that girl once and I felt bad for her.

Sitting there as the professor passed out the exam, I thought about Jason. I'd met him during that freshman summer bridge program. The three-year age gap might as well have been 10, given my limited dating experience. Jason was mahogany colored with captivating bronze eyes and a sculpted physique. He was well dressed, confident, and charming. He was in school but also worked full-time at an automotive plant. He had an apartment off campus. I ignored the rest of the red flags.

My new college friends frequently proposed makeovers to improve my hairstyle, encourage makeup experimentation, and convince me to upgrade my wardrobe from my rural attire. Once content with the outcome, they cheerfully nudged me down the hallway, hoping to catch Jason's attention.

I harbored doubts about their plan. Boys seldom noticed me in high school, so I remained skeptical about its potential success. However, to my astonishment, it worked. He asked for my phone number. I was in a situation I hadn't prepared for, unsure of how to proceed. So, I did nothing. Well, remarkably little. I devoted much of my time and attention to Jason.

I discounted his pathological lies and ignored his chronic "borrowing." His electricity got shut off. He was short on rent. He didn't have food. I loaned him money from my school refund check. I let him use my campus food card. He never paid me back and bought food for other people on my card. He was supposed to keep the moving truck filled with our dorm furniture safe at his place overnight. He told me it had gotten robbed, but I noticed the lock wasn't broken. My friend found my stereo in his friend's room months later.

At the start, though, I thought I was in love. I skipped morning classes. I didn't do my weekly readings or go to study tables. I crammed for exams. Then, I had the nerve to be surprised when I got B's and C's. I cried over the D, college algebra. I blamed it on the professor's accent instead of my absences.

By the mid-spring of my first year, when Jason broke up with me, I was more relieved than heartbroken, but the damage to my life was done. My Fall semester GPA had dropped in half, cutting my overall score to 2.6. My structure was all but gone. I failed to realize that it was a structure that got me all As the prior summer. I had failed. I was now "the person on your left or right."

Losing focus for a moment cost me a $1,000 academic book scholarship. Had I gotten 0.1 more, I would've been safe with a 2.0. Also, I would've been safe from the bridge program director calling my grandparents.

I picked up the receiver of the green corded phone in my dorm before my roommate, Elizabeth.

"Bridgette, it's Granny. Pawpaw is on the line." A stone hit the bottom of my stomach. Commonly, Granny called me "Bridge," and we talked on Sunday nights. She'd used my full name; it was the middle of the week. Trouble.

"What are you doing up there? We got a call from a lady saying you were messing up in school." The scary version of Pawpaw's voice came through the line.

"You didn't go up there to be chasing after some knuckleheaded boy. You went for school! You need to get your priorities straight."

"I'll do better." It was all I could say as the tears pooled in my eyes. I'd let them down. I'd been like my mother and got caught up with a man, a no-good one at that. I'd messed up my money, lending it to Jason as if I had any to spare. It would take a miracle to recover my grades. I knew I'd messed up, but now I was embarrassed. They knew.

The load of my family weighed heavily on me. I was the first to go to college. My grandparents half-joked that I'd one day buy Pawpaw a Porsche and Granny a bright yellow Jeep, her dream car when I was a success. It felt like they'd pinned their hopes and dreams on me, and I was carrying theirs along with mine. If I failed, we all failed. That was the weight of poverty.

It was the reality check that I needed. Even after Jason and I briefly reconciled for the summer, school became my first and foremost priority. I studied immediately after class and skipped naps and socializing until my work was finished. I got an on-campus work-study job with Student Services that allowed me to do schoolwork in my downtime. For the longest, I thought the phrasing "work-study" was literal and applied to all campus jobs. I was so naïve, but learning. To get my books, I took out loans from the library, found old editions of textbooks, and photocopied other people's materials. I was hustling to repair the damage. And it worked. Only it wasn't retroactive.

After seven semesters of near perfection, I recovered one point on my GPA. I graduated college cum laude (3.6) with distinction…and disappointment. I learned a lot on the way; most importantly, I didn't want to be a lawyer.

Focusing back on my policing final, I aced it with ease. I'd finished the criminal justice major, but I'd started on an entirely new plan a year earlier in my senior year. I was no longer distracted.

References

1. Finch, K., Lawrence, D., Williams, M. O., Thompson, A. R., & Hartwright, C. (2024). Relationships between adverse childhood experiences, attachment, resilience, psychological distress and trauma among forensic mental health populations. *The Journal of Forensic Psychiatry & Psychology*, *35*(5), 660–684. https://doi.org/10.1080/14789949.2024.2365149
2. Benton, S. (2017). *The savior complex: Why good intentions may have negative outcomes.* Psychology Today. https://www.psychologytoday.com/us/blog/the-high-functioning-alcoholic/201702/the-savior-complex

CHAPTER 8

You Have the Right to Remain Silent

Adverse Childhood Experiences and Adult Patterns

ACEs can influence the relationships and environments we gravitate toward in adulthood. This unconscious repetition of familiar dynamics often perpetuates cycles of trauma and dysfunction.[1]

IN MY JUNIOR year of college, I became enamored with Dr. Vaughn. Dr. V wore her box braids down to her thin waist. She was petite but filled the room when she entered.

"Most of you WILL fail this class," she'd bellow in her deep voice, rolling her neck and eyes with a Nigerian attitude. I planned to prove her wrong, but my stomach wavered. I couldn't afford to fail...again.

There were many more open seats on the second day of her class. Then, Dr. V revealed that she had intended to "weed out the weak" with her speech. My ears heard, "You are strong," and my shoulders released. I could do this.

Dr. V entertained us with tales of being the "Black Dollar Tree Princess of Connecticut." Her immigrant father owned five stores. She'd gone to college at 16 and graduated with honors. She was "one of five Black women in the entire country with dual doctorates." And men bowed at her feet, or so she'd tell me later.

A group of us gathered to talk to Dr. V after every class. I emailed her with questions about the assignments. We stood in line like fans, patiently waiting to meet with her during her office hours. She never rushed us. She leaned back in her chair and gossiped like a girlfriend. Within a month, I'd earned VIP tickets to her house. There was only one problem. I had no car, and the bus didn't go near her condo. I averted my eyes as I shared my plight with Dr. V.

"You can ride with me," Dr. V offered.

Be cool, Bridgette. Be cool. "OK, that sounds good," my voice cracked a bit. It felt like I was a V in VIP.

(dis)Honor Thy Mother: Daughterhood, Dysfunction and Deliverance, First Edition. Bridgette Peteet.
© 2026 John Wiley & Sons, Inc. Published 2026 by John Wiley & Sons, Inc.

After the next class, Dr. V and I walked out of the lecture hall toward the adjacent parking lot. We approached a strange vehicle that seemed the polar opposite of the tiny red sports car I'd seen the department chair drag himself out of some mornings. Dr. V's car reminded me of my first car, a 1978 Chevy Nova, but in blue.

The door on my side was jammed, so Dr. V climbed in and pushed it open from the driver's side. Papers, fast food wrappers, and random pieces of clothing covered the seats in front and back. She shoved the trash to the side and told me to get in. Dog odors and white hair wafted from the seat as I sat down, balancing my purse and book bag on my knees and not touching anything.

To my surprise, people were already inside Dr. V's townhouse when we arrived. Familiar faces of staff and campus acquaintances greeted me with curiosity. The perimeter of Dr. V's living room mirrored the scene in her car. Surfaces had been cleared so that we could sit, but the contents had been pushed onto the floor nearby.

One perpetually grumpy staff member turned from making snacks to grunting a hello in my direction. The rebound frat guy from that policing final was there, too. He seemed completely comfortable, as if he'd been there many times. I sat on the edge of the couch, trying not to take up too much space or touch anything. We ate taco salad and socialized. Dr. V asked about our hopes and dreams and encouraged us to dream bigger. I asked for a ride home from another student. We left late into the evening. The rebound guy did not.

The format of Dr. V's class dimmed my law school dreams even more. It was tedious. Did the nine Chief Justices take 4,759 words to say "yes" or "no"? I'd nod off, trying to memorize case laws just enough to scribble down the contents in my blue book for an exam before gratefully forgetting everything I'd read.

"This is what law school is like," Dr. V suggested afterward with pride, while I mentally hurled.

That same semester, I was taking my general education requirements and enrolled in abnormal psychology. It was my second psychology class. Psych 101 had given me a basic overview of different parts of the field, but this? This class was a revelation. There seemed to be a light around the professor as she educated us about a myriad of mental illnesses.

You mean to tell me there's a name for this stuff! I leaned in from the edge of my seat in the giant lecture hall.

The professor had advised us not to try to diagnose ourselves or others based on what we learned. We weren't qualified. Still, it was hard to resist.

That explains it.

I'm not crazy.

So and so needs help.

What my family called sadness, laziness, eccentricity, odd thinking, or the effects of a spiked drink were actually depression, personality disorders, and bipolar disease. I was like a sponge, digesting every word assigned to us and hanging on to my professor's every utterance. She went on to tell us that there were also treatment options for these illnesses. Sign me up!

I was hooked. But, I had no "hook-up" in psychology. I had no idea what steps to take besides declaring it as my second major.

I shared my dilemma over coffee one morning with Dr. V.

"Since you don't want to attend law school, have you considered getting your PhD in psychology?" Dr. V asked. "You can go to graduate school instead of law school!" she said excitedly as if she'd just figured out my life for me.

I had to be honest. I had no idea what graduate school was. I'd heard of "getting a Master's" but didn't know what it meant. Dr. V explained it all to me. There was a third option besides medical or law school to continue my education. If I went all the way, I could become a different kind of doctor, a Ph.D.

"How do I do that?"

Dr. V told me to meet with a faculty advisor in psychology. Dr. Herman's afro gave me a false sense of comfort and familiarity as I sat across from him.

"I want to get my Ph.D in psychology," I shared proudly to the tall Jewish man sitting behind his desk. I thought he'd be impressed with my ambition. He wasn't.

"Getting into a Ph.D in psychology is extremely difficult, more challenging than medical school. Programs take incredibly few students."

"Do you want to know my GPA?" I said, continuing with slightly less self-assurance.

Dr. Herman nodded.

"A 3.4."

Dr. Herman's eyebrows raised. He bobbed his head up and down, and his lips pressed together. "That's decent, but it's still not good enough. Have you considered a career in social work?"

I slumped in my chair. I hadn't thought of it. I briefly considered what I knew of the career. Women removing children from their homes like we had been five years earlier? No, thank you. Dr. Herman gave me the chair's name in the Department of Social Work and waved me toward the door.

"Really quickly, can you tell me what else I need to do to make myself more competitive in psychology?" I'd had my notepad ready to go. In that freshman summer bridge program, I'd learned always to take paper and pen to meetings.

Dr. Herman half rolled his eyes before rattling off a list—research experience, three strong letters from professors, a personal statement, a CV, teaching experience, clinical experience, and good GRE scores.

The crooked letters of my scribbles stared back at me, that "terrible penmanship" my mother loathed. I stepped out of Dr. Herman's office and into the hallway. I was working in Dr. V's research lab by then. She would write me a letter. That's one. What was a "CV?" The GRE sounded like a test. I'd heard of the MCAT and the LSAT. I thought the LSAT covered everything that wasn't related to medicine. Guess not.

I swiped my tears away as I trudged back to my dorm, thinking there was no way I could do this.

"You've got this," Dr. V sat unblinking at her desk as I finished relaying the long list to her.

"You can be my teaching assistant, and we'll get you connected with another research lab in psychology. I'll write you a letter, and that new mentor will too."

I went to meet with the Chair of the Department of Social Work. He'd dismissed me quickly after learning I wanted to be a clinician, not a professor. I also met with the Dean of the Honor's College at Dr. B's encouragement.

"How'd we let you slip through the cracks?" he asked as his eyes widened and his brow creased in surprise at my academic performance. The Dean allowed me to switch my research hours to the honors level. I'd complete a senior thesis and graduate with an additional honors designation.

The rest of the Spring semester of junior year and the fall of my senior year were a whirlwind. I took 21 credit hours to acquire all the psychology courses I needed to apply for graduate school. I'd added psychology on top of my criminal justice major. I did research. I volunteered as a peer mentor and facilitated groups for prospective freshman and their parents. I got a job over the Christmas break as support staff for adult men with disabilities. I was a teaching assistant again. I bought a used GRE prep book and started studying.

Dr. V connected me with a senior professor in psychology. I started working in "Dr. Angela's" lab that fall. She seemed like the tame version of Dr. V. She was measured, well-respected, and got things done. Though I didn't know it, I gained a new mentor just in time to lose the old.

Dr. V was on a rampage in her office one morning. The department was going to fire her. That was my simplistic understanding of the situation. My stomach tightened. She told me that her Chair said she "wrote like an early career graduate student" and that her teaching evaluations were poor. They stated that her classes were "too hard" because she structured her undergraduate classes like law school when most of us wouldn't go beyond our bachelor's degree.

Dr. V showed me an email stream that had been circulated amongst the faculty in the department. It started with a fake test with questions like "If Tyriq has 13 Glocks and sells 5 to Jamal, how many does he have left?"

One faculty member in the chain suggested it should be the exit exam for students in the major because it might help boost our scores. It was sickening to know what they secretly thought about the diversity of students in our major.

Racism was apparent in the classroom as well. Some students commented, "Black people commit more crime" and "Justice is blind to color," which directly contradicted the research studies we were reading. Dr. V didn't let it slide and taught us to frame our arguments with evidence rather than emotion. I couldn't do it and the heated debates left me angry and depleted. I imagined that those with opposing arguments also expressed their frustrations with Dr. V's course evaluations. I felt like we needed to defend her, but how?

Dr. V suggested that I organize a protest on her behalf. I was not the demonstration type, flying under the radar and avoiding trouble. I'd seen images of protesters getting arrested, and I was scared. Thanks to my courses, I knew too well what happened once you got sucked into the justice system. Sensing my resistance, Dr. V suggested a silent, anonymous protest.

Pretending to have a team of organizers, I got to work. The black-and-white flyers said, "Fight Racism. Stop the Firing of our Only Black Professor. Silent Protest. Wear All Black," announcing the date and time of the event. I passed the flyers out in classes and posted them around the department. When students asked me questions, I told them what "we" were trying to do. Several students offered to help distribute the flyers. I called the campus newspaper, made an anonymous report about the department emails, and provided the protest details. It was all coming together, but I worried no one would attend.

The afternoon of the protest, I entered the main level of the criminal justice building. I was relieved to see two dozen or more protesters lining the hallways. Students of all races wore black and stood silently along the walls. Some had handmade signs saying, "Save Dr. V!" I walked to the end of one line and stood as if I were a regular participant.

Meeting attendees trailed into the conference room. I recognized the department chair and a few of my professors, who glanced at us as they passed. My stomach clenched. A few moments later, at the other end of the hall, Dr. V entered the double doors of the building flanked by men with briefcases. She scanned the crowd, and the corners of her eyes creased in approval. My nerves subsided. I'd done well.

As we waited, a reporter moved down the line, trying to get someone to talk. "Who organized this?" No one answered. A white guy from one of my classes pointed at me. My body tensed again. The reporter approached me with a pencil and notepad in hand.

"Did you organize this?"

"Several students organized this event," I lied.

"What's your name?"

"This is an anonymous protest. Students here fear retaliation from the department and don't want to be identified."

"I can quote you without your name. Would that be okay?"

Out of excuses, I agreed.

"What's this protest about?"

I nervously elaborated on the points outlined in the flyer and answered a few of her follow-up questions. Once satisfied, she stood beside us and waited for the meeting to end.

More than an hour later, the conference room doors broke the hall's silence. Those who had taken a seat on the floor to rest stood up. Our necks strained, searching the scene for an answer. No one met our eyes. Dr. V turned away from us and left the building. Professors and administrators filed out in turn.

Once they were gone, someone whispered, "What do we do next?" People started looking in my direction. I had no idea what we were supposed to do. This was the end of her plan.

"I guess that's it," I offered in reluctant leadership.

The following week, I lamented about the firing of Dr. V to one of our deans. He was the only Black administrator on campus at the time. He nodded intermittently as I spoke but said little in response. I could tell he was holding back. When I finished, he leaned forward on his desk and folded his hands thoughtfully as if figuring out how to say what he wanted. He stated simply and supportively, "You don't know all of it."

My body jolted to attention. I knew exactly, well almost exactly, what he meant. He'd said even more than he realized. I'd only heard Dr. V's version of events. I didn't search for other information. I overlooked the signs that there could be other issues—stories that didn't add up, few boundaries, questionable relationships, braggadociousness, blaming others, never taking accountability. I knew this personality type.

Dr. V was just like Mom. That revelation shook me to my core. I'd replicated the unhealthy mother–daughter dynamics with a pseudo-surrogate mother. Consciously, I hated this personality style. Subconsciously, it was familiar, and I was somehow drawn to it. This is likely because in the relationship with Dr. V, I got to be the golden child. The pet that believed she could do no wrong. It was a euphoric feeling compared to the scapegoat role I was used to in my family. Whether privileged or disadvantaged positions, all roads fulfill a pathological need for control and validation within this type of person.

Like Mom, I thought I could save Dr. V, but I could not save them from themselves. It took me a long time to realize I only had one life preserver. I'd sink trying to rescue others with that limited resource. I needed a boat if I was going to help more people.

***

My new mentor in psychology, Dr. Angela, invited me to a two-day weekend admission boot camp with eight other Black psychology majors in the Fall of my senior year. We learned that the acceptance rate for Ph.D programs was in the single digits. We turned our resumes into CVs, a curriculum vitae summarizing our academic skills and experiences. We created rough drafts of one-page, single-spaced personal statements telling our stories, career aspirations, research activities, and interests. Admissions applications were due for the following Fall term at the end of the calendar year.

On our last lunch break of the weekend, one of the participants turned to me and shared, "There's *no* way to finish all of this. I'm just going to wait until next year." I understood her position. Even after all I'd done to get on the right track for graduate school, the finish line felt so far away.

I shrugged. "We might as well try since the odds of getting in are so low." But the girl had already turned away from me.

Another statistic swirled in my head. Most people who took a gap year between college and graduate school didn't apply later. I didn't want to fall into the gap. With nothing to lose, I continued forward. I was the only one from the entire program.

Dr. Angela became my grad school coach. We met every week. She helped me identify my research interests. She suggested five to six psychology doctoral programs to apply to in the state. She read drafts and drafts of my CV and personal statement. That effort, along with taking 21 credit hours, had me stressed. I was only slightly relieved once all of the applications were submitted. I'd have to wait more than a month to hear any news.

The envelopes started coming in in early February. These letters weren't like the ones I had collected in high school. None of them were shiny or thick. Thin envelopes with a single piece of paper inside clung to the sides of my metal mailbox every few days. Rejections.

"Dear Bridgette. We regret to inform you…"

Do you "regret" it though? My hopes sank with each one.

I got a second letter from Bowling Green State University.

Did they change their minds? I opened the seal optimistically.

"Dear Bridgette. We regret to inform you…"

Seriously? I crumpled that one up and slam-dunked it into the trash on the way to the cafeteria. I consoled myself with breadsticks and marinara.

Later that week, I got a phone call in my dorm. It was someone named Dr. Burlew from the University of Cincinnati (UC). I hadn't listed her as a potential mentor in my personal statement, but she wanted to know if I'd like to come and interview with her anyway.

"YES," I shouted before she could finish speaking. I covered my mouth to conceal my enthusiasm. *Be cool, Bridgette. Be cool.*

Ultimately, UC was my only interview invitation.

Over the next couple of weeks, Dr. Angela's preparation revved up. I met with her twice a week. Wear this, don't wear that. Drive this, don't ride that. Drink this, don't drink that. Ask this, don't ask that. Say this, don't say that. Some of it seemed silly to me. Would they care if I took the Greyhound bus instead of renting a car? I doubted it but listened to her anyway.

I bought my first adult suit that wasn't from the junior's department. It had a skirt and pants that I could rotate to get me through the grueling two-day interview schedule. I rented the cheapest car I could find. When I arrived at UC's campus, I asked the right questions. I flailed with some of my answers and did fine on others. When the graduate students took us out for a social, I declined alcohol while other applicants didn't. Overall, I had no idea how I'd done.

The stress of it all made me sick. I couldn't drive four hours back to campus, so I stopped in my hometown halfway between. Granny nursed me back to health overnight, and I got back on the road the following day.

A week later, I heard my phone ringing from my dorm hallway. I sprinted for the receiver and picked it up before my answering machine did.

"Hello!" I said breathlessly.

"May I speak to Bridgette?"

"This is she."

"This is Dr. Burlew from UC. How are you?"

"Fine," I answered, but wasn't. Where had all of the air gone in the room? Was it hot in here?

"I'm calling to offer you a position in our psychology doctoral program this fall."

My legs gave out, and my knees hit a thin rug covering my room's tiled floor.

"YES, YES, YES!" I shrieked into the receiver before remembering Dr. Angela's coaching.

"Um, yes, that sounds good, Dr. Burlew. I'd be happy to attend this fall. Thank you so much for the invitation."

We made a follow-up plan, said our farewells, and hung up. I rocked back and forth on my knees, tears of joy springing from my eyes. I couldn't believe it. It had been a year since I'd learned what graduate school was, and now I was going. I would get a masters and Ph.D all at once. A bigger life preserver. Maybe a boat.

The air practically buzzed excitedly as I shared the details with friends and family. The genuine joy in their voices mirrored the happiness that was bubbling within me. Everyone was proud—almost everyone.

***

She was 50, white, with silver roots pushing through dyed blonde hair and a look in her eyes that told me she'd been doing life on her own for a very long time. We'll call her *Lynn*. She arrived early for every session, sat stiffly on the couch, and made direct eye contact only when she was being sarcastic.

"I'm just not good with people," she said flatly one day, brushing invisible lint from her jeans. "I try, but something always happens. They do one thing wrong and then I ghost. I know I do it. I just…can't seem to stop."

It didn't take long to connect the dots. Lynn had a long history of adverse childhood experiences: physical neglect, parental substance use, and the ever-present emotional unavailability of a mother who saw vulnerability as weakness. She had learned early that needing people came with a price. And the cost was often too high to bear.

Lynn spoke in scattered fragments about her past, as if flipping through old, damaged photos she didn't really want to look at. "My mom wasn't mean," she insisted. "She just. . .wasn't interested. In me. In my feelings. I'd come home from school crying and she'd say, 'Well, what did *you* do to make them treat you like that?' "

She laughed, bitterly. "You learn not to cry after a while."

I nodded, gently. "It makes sense," I said. "If the people who were supposed to comfort you made you feel like a burden, your brain learned to keep people out. Not because you don't care, but because connection didn't feel safe."

Lynn looked at me then, long and hard. "So you're saying I'm not broken?"

"Not at all," I said. "You did what it needed to survive in your childhood. But the problem is that those same survival strategies, like withdrawing or avoiding closeness, can backfire in adulthood. Especially when you *do* want connection. We repeat our childhood patterns with others."

I explained how avoidant attachment patterns often grow out of emotionally neglectful or dismissive early environments and affect our adult social interactions.[2,3] As children, people like Lynn learn that emotions are unwelcome, that vulnerability leads to shame, and that it's safer to depend on oneself. They build protective walls. They report higher negative affect, stress, and experiences of social rejection.[3] But those same walls later become prisons, keeping others out and also keeping their own needs locked in.

"It's not that you're incapable of connection," I told her. "It's that you don't *trust* it yet. And that's something we can work on."

We spent sessions identifying her triggers—moments when she felt overwhelmed by closeness or expectations—and developing strategies to pause before retreating. We practiced noticing the urge to run and sitting with the discomfort instead of running from it.

"It's weird," she said months later. "I had coffee with a woman from work. She said something irritating. When I started to feel the panic rise, like, 'this is getting too real,' I heard your voice. Telling me to breathe. That I could stay. That it was just my past showing up in the present."

Lynn was still figuring it out. She still struggled with interpersonal relationships and still felt safest when she was the one giving help, not receiving it. But she was trying.

References

1. Lebow, H. I. (2021). *How childhood trauma may affect adult relationships.* PsychCentral. https://psychcentral.com/blog/how-childhood-trauma-affects-adult-relationships#what-is-childhood-trauma

2. Bowlby, J. (1973). *Separation: Anxiety and anger. Attachment and loss* (Vol. 2). New York, NY: Basic Books.

3. Sheinbaum, T., Kwapil, T. R., Ballespí, S., Mitjavila, M., Chun, C. A., Silvia, P. J., … Barrantes-Vidal, N. (2015). Attachment style predicts affect, cognitive appraisals, and social functioning in daily life. *Frontiers in Psychology, 6,* 296.

CHAPTER 9

Love and War

Adverse Childhood Experience—Domestic Violence

Domestic violence is an ACE when a child witnesses violence in the home or community.[1]

THE AIR IN Cincinnati felt somehow thicker than the other parts of the state where I'd grown up and gone to college. The rolling acres of green grass I was used to were replaced with never-ending hills of concrete. It was odd for a city in the Midwest that Cincinnatians seemed startled by annual snowfalls. The city was almost half Black but there was no shared familiarity of growing up together or collectivistic head nods that said "I see you" as you walked across campus. Instead, students walked with their eyes averted downwards, headphones on, assuring our anonymity and isolation. Grown people in the city "repped" their high schools as if they'd graduated yesterday instead of one, two, or three decades prior. Every tenth block was a different neighborhood designation. Additions like "North" or "East" subtly signaled that one community was better than its fraternal twin. There was this invisible line between the university and the surrounding neighborhood that few dared cross. I didn't fit on either side.

I was 22 and looking for my first apartment in a major city. With no credit history, prospective landlords rejected me repeatedly. I needed a co-signer. I had no one to ask and was growing weary in my search for housing. As with everything, I told my grandparents what was going on. I prayed they would take pity and offer help, but I would never directly ask. I didn't want to be a burden to anyone. I wanted people to see that I was responsible and offer to help out of their own free will. They didn't. My grandparents took the rare opportunity to demonstrate fiscal responsibility and boundary-setting. I couldn't blame them. Too often they gave more than they could afford to other relatives, which cost them regularly.

At the time, I didn't understand. Later, I'd go on to adopt the same policy. No co-signing. I might have to revise that when my children get older, but so far that's the rule. At that moment, my grandparents' limits felt inconsistent. I respected their decision because I could accept boundaries. I hadn't yet learned though to create them for myself.

I was growing more and more hopeless at each apartment building. About to be dismissed again, I pleaded with one leasing agent to give me a chance. She flippantly mentioned an exception for applicants with more than $5,000 in their checking account as if it were irrelevant to me. My eyes glistened. I had $9,000 in savings thanks to my full-time summer job.

I rented the bottom floor, two-bedroom apartment for $420 of my upcoming $800 monthly graduate student stipend. After deposits, I planned to supplement my income with my savings over the next year. I paid my rent on time every time. In my mind, I was proving the doubters wrong. On the other hand, I didn't always have money for groceries. Eating probably should have been a priority, but I was "full" of pride that my debts were paid.

Hunger eventually got the best of me, and someone suggested I apply for an electronic benefit transfer (EBT) card. Even though I'd grown up with limited resources, I didn't know anything about the complexities of the welfare system. My mother used to say, "Welfare is for people who don't work." She had more pride than ethics, though, as she had no issues buying food stamps from her patients at the clinic for $0.50 on the dollar. My dad and most of his family were better off, but my siblings and I rarely reaped the benefits. Dad had biweekly visitation and would otherwise say, "You all only call when you need something." I'd think *if only he knew how much we needed and didn't ask.*

I headed downtown to the county family services office and lined up outside. I wasn't even sure I was in the right place, so I asked the young woman before me. In college, I learned my lesson about waiting in the wrong queue for campus services. The young woman confirmed that I was in the right place and spent the next hour wrestling her two young children into quiet submission.

When it was my turn, I approached the counter with a smile. The worker already looked like she was having a horrendous day. She was middle-aged and wearing chained reading glasses.

"I'd like to apply for an EBT card, please," I proclaimed and handed her my application.

She glanced at the front page and asked about my employment.

"I don't have a job, but I'm in graduate school getting my Ph.D."

It was a simple case of a poor, hungry student struggling to survive and make a better life. It seemed to be just what the system wanted. I thought she'd be impressed with me as the ideal candidate. Instead, she slid her glasses down her nose and gave me a distasteful glare.

"Doctoral students don't qualify for benefits," she retorted coolly.

That was it. She sent me away, seemingly relieved to clear someone from her line. Years later, I realized the decision should have been based on my income, but I accepted her word and didn't fight. I held back tears as I rushed to my car, parked at a meter a few blocks away. I figured it was best for a country girl not to appear vulnerable and cry in the city's downtown streets.

I had no idea where I'd gone wrong. Fortunately, I did know how to deal with hunger. Drink a large glass of water, go to bed early to stave off the hunger pangs, and pray that I didn't wake up in the middle of the night.

***

It took me a minute to adapt to nighttime in the city. The sirens and traffic zipping up Queen City Avenue differed from the crickets and wind I was used to hearing when night settled in. On my first evening in my new apartment, I'd asked a neighborhood boy for directions to the nearest grocery store. He seemed concerned that I planned to go there alone—at night. I assured him of my 'grownness' and set off. The dimly lit parking lot full of questionable characters, the dingy tile of the store floor, and the creepy guy who refused to take "no" for an answer when he asked for my phone number in the checkout line had confirmed his concern. I ultimately found another store a bit further away. Same chain, better neighborhood.

That weekend, my dad and cousin drove the rest of my stuff down in my dad's pick-up truck. Tony Sr. got out and immediately commented on my surroundings.

"Why'd you move to the hood?" his nose raised.

I looked around. Did this count as the hood? Being from a small town I wasn't sure. I didn't see any graffiti, gangs, or garbage as depicted in movies about life in the ghetto. Maybe I was "hood adjacent?" I'd been warned about the imaginary street boundaries between "safe" and "unsafe" neighborhoods in Cincinnati. If so, there was nothing that I could do. It was what I could afford and I had a year-long lease.

Dad continued his interrogation.

"Why'd you get an apartment on the first floor?"

He'd lobbed this question over his shoulder as he carried an oversized box down the stairs to my unit on the left.

Wait. Was that a bad thing? It had seemed ideal. The first floor was cheaper. As a bonus, downstairs meant that it was easier to move things in. It was benefiting him right at this moment. So, what was wrong with the first floor? What was he talking about? Maybe with his background in construction, Dad was worried about structural issues. Yes, that must be it. With my parents, it often felt better not to ask questions and try to figure it out alone. Sometimes I made mistakes.

A week before classes started, I walked into my kitchen to make a phone call. I picked up the receiver off the wall—no dial tone. I repeatedly pressed the switch hook. Silence. As I stood there, the sheetrock began to turn gray, and a pool of water began to drizzle onto the edge between the tile and the carpet of the living room. I looked at my kitchen sink. It was off. It must be coming from upstairs.

I rushed beast mode up the stairs to the apartment above me. After banging on the door for a few moments, a petite and groggy African woman came to the door. I pointed to her kitchen and sink as she stood alone, sopping wet floors in a haze. She'd turned the sink on and had fallen asleep.

With empathy, I sensed her exhaustion. I'd heard her two young children playing every day above my head. At night, I'd often heard the sounds of her husband's fists as he pounded her to the floor. I called the police every time. I would longer be the child hiding in the bathroom, fearing the violent sounds of my parents' fighting seeping under the door. I had power.

One sunny afternoon months later, the husband from upstairs stopped me in the entryway of our building. I was retrieving my mail from the communal golden boxes on the landing. He was a short, slight African man with bulging eyes.

"I know it's you that keep calling the police on me," he sneered in broken English and a thick accent.

I wanted to say something smart-alecky like, "Maybe don't beat your wife, and I won't have to call the police," but I didn't want to take my chances. He said nothing more, so I sidestepped him and retreated to my apartment at a pace that feigned confidence.

The neighbor's wife eventually kicked him out, but I knew from life experience and now textbooks that didn't always last. Years later, I saw her across the aisles of a department store. I expected her to look away like she usually did when I'd passed her in our building. Instead, she gave me the faintest nod and smile as if to say she was okay.

***

Back in that first apartment, my neighbor problems continued. Two college-age men lived directly across from me, and one beat up his girlfriend one winter night. She'd escaped when he went to the bathroom and banged on my door. I won't lie; I didn't want to let her in. I didn't know her. She didn't live in our building. Why didn't she run out the front door? Here, in my apartment, he could easily follow.

Through my peephole, her distorted face appeared frantic. I knew I had no choice. I let her in and slammed my door closed just as his opened, and he charged across the hall. My hands shook as I twisted the lock and deadbolt and secured the chain as he reached the door. Unlike my other upstairs neighbor, this guy was massive. The security measures didn't seem strong enough as my door rattled under his blows. The stranger and I huddled together on my couch in tears until the police arrived. I took great pleasure watching through the peephole as two small female officers hog-tied his hands and feet together before I opened the door. I never saw him again.

***

April of 2001 brought civil unrest to the downtown streets of Cincinnati. Protestors took to the streets in response to a police officer killing an unarmed Black man, Timothy Thomas, and other injustices. Helicopters whirred overhead. Videos of events circulated on the news day and night, seemingly intent on scaring us. I was afraid until I saw the pattern and recognized that it was the same four images on repeat. An overturned hot dog stand. Two trash cans were knocked over. A protester throwing a soda can at the police. A motorist was pulled from their car and assaulted. Not to minimize a violent act, but how were any of these images more distressing than a shooting? Someone had died. That should be the focus.

A supposed 8 p.m.–6 a.m. citywide curfew was enacted but only enforced in specific "diverse" neighborhoods. Life in the city was draining to me. The breaking point came soon.

I was praying next to my bed one night in late September. The world's troubles, including the 9/11 attacks and surviving graduate school, weighed heavily on me. I got off my knees and flipped off my light simultaneously, revealing the shadow of a man peeping through my bedroom window. I clutched my chest and screamed. The figure stood up and ran away. I grabbed my phone and crawled into the hallway, where there were no windows. I frantically dialed my boyfriend, now husband, and whispered that a man was outside and he needed to come over right away.

I sat quivering and silently waiting so the man outside wouldn't know where I was in the apartment. I listened for windows rattling or breaking but heard nothing except my heartbeat. Afraid that he would hear me talking, I didn't make a second call to the police. The next day, I told the property manager I was moving and wanted my full deposit back.

"Why would you get an apartment on the first floor anyway?" she asked.

This time, I knew the answer to this persistent question. I felt dumb that I didn't know in the first place. It was more evidence of my lack of street smarts. But even my supposed book smarts seemed to be failing me, too.

Reference

1. Centers for Disease Control (CDC). (n.d.). *Fast facts: Preventing adverse childhood experiences.* https://www.cdc.gov/violenceprevention/aces/fastfact.html

CHAPTER 10

If It Were Easy, Everyone Would Do It

<u>Impostorism</u>

Impostor syndrome, is the persistent belief that your achievements are undeserved and that you're a fraud waiting to be exposed.[1]

DR. BURLEW, my graduate school mentor, had some news. She smiled as she told me I would deliver a lecture during the third week of her *Introduction to Psychology* class while she was away for a research conference. I was her teaching assistant (TA) and had been in graduate school for seven days. My soul left my body.

"I graduated college five months ago. I was just on their level."

"No. They're mostly freshman. You have four years more of school than them, and you have your degree."

Dr. Burlew had a point.

"Also, think about where you'll be in four years. Is it the same as where you are now?"

In that time, I would be finishing my graduate degree. That discrepancy was a helpful reality check. I had a long way to go but had also come so far.

Dr. Burlew had a way of seeing things I didn't see in myself. I thought graduating would be a miracle, but she believed I would do so much more. I looked up to her, literally and figuratively. She was tall with a friendly face. She was twenty years into her tenure, spending most of her time as the only Black woman on the faculty. She was a reserved powerhouse. She didn't brag about her many academic and research accomplishments. She worked because she cared about the people she studied. She showed concern about the students in her lab and their personal and professional well-being. I imprinted on her like a baby duckling, following her lead. Dr. Burlew became my academic mother. This time, I chose right.

(dis)Honor Thy Mother: Daughterhood, Dysfunction and Deliverance, First Edition. Bridgette Peteet.
© 2026 John Wiley & Sons, Inc. Published 2026 by John Wiley & Sons, Inc.

Her encouragement boosted my confidence by about 22% (pause for nerd humor). I conceded. I was teaching 223 students in two weeks. She said it would be simple. All I had to do was prepare and review a slide deck for half of the class and show a video for the remainder of the time. Simple. For her, yes. For me? My slight nervousness at public speaking became a full-blown panic.

Time began fast-forwarding, and I found myself hyper-focused, going down the long steps of the giant lecture hall, trying to remember how to walk and praying that I didn't fall. My heart was thumping in my ears. My stomach growled because I skipped breakfast like usual. I made it to the oversized lectern and started pushing the appropriate buttons to rev up the computer and projector. I held my breath as hundreds of students filed into their seats. They were probably used to seeing me set up before taking my seat as the TA. Today, I dressed up and didn't sit down with them. My mouth was dry. My Secret deodorant was telling on me. I imagined them realizing that I was lecturing and wishing they'd skipped class that day. It was 9:00 a.m. on the dot.

"Dr. Burlew is out for a conference today, and I'll be lecturing. I'm your TA, Bridgette."

A two-note catcall came from the top of the lecture hall; the one men do to show interest in a woman, simultaneously it objectified me and degraded my authority. A few giggles sprinkled throughout the crowd while most faces waited expectantly before starting to blur. My spine gave out a little. My cheeks were on fire.

I'd worn my graduate school interview suit to class that day, dressing up so the students would take me seriously. My hair was pulled back in the low, short ponytail I'd wear for the next five school years. My face was bare because that's what "serious" academics did. I looked the part. Smart. Serious.

I'd rehearsed and written down every word I would say, even my name. I was worried I'd forget it. I'd studied the chapter like I was the one who would be tested so that I could answer any questions the students might have. When I readied my mental list of catastrophies, I'd anticipated a student asking me a question I didn't know the answer to, technology failing, or completely blanking out and forgetting what to say. I had a mental plan for those. I'd get back to a student with the answer, call IT for help with the computer, and read from the slides. I could read. I'd always been exceptional at reading. But, a catcall? It hadn't crossed my mind. No one had prepared me for it. No one could have prepared me for it.

Too much time had passed in silence. How would a professor respond? I didn't know. Maybe they would correct the student. But who? I wasn't sure where the sound had originated. How would I react on the street? I'd cringe and ignore it. Good plan. I clicked past the title slide and started talking.

In 17 minutes, I was finished. I checked the clock at the back of the hall uncomfortably. It was supposed to be 30 minutes, half of the class. Breathe. Two hundred eyes blinked down at me, cartoon smoke billowing from their pens as they tried to keep pace. Breathe. Their faces started to blur again. Breathe. My eyes landed on the encased video. Breathe. I squatted down behind the podium where the students couldn't see me and fumbled with the VHS tape, *Learning*. Breathe. The outdated video appeared on the three screens high above my head. I stalled, pretending it still needed my attention, hiding out of sight for several moments longer, breathing, and vowing *never* to become a professor.

***

Graduate school was not the next level of education. It felt like it had skipped ahead 3–4 steps. Each quarter, we took 4–5 classes in 3-hour blocks each. We were TAs for up to 10 hours a week. We were research assistants for another 10 hours. We had between 5 and 20 hours of clinical practicums, depending on our year in the program. That did not include our academic milestones, including two qualifying exams, a master's thesis, and a dissertation.

For the entire first year of training, I scribbled feverishly in my notebooks until my wrists hurt and my eyes watered, hoping I'd caught most of the lesson. I can recall my indignation when one instructor informed us that the average human attention span is 30–45 minutes. It felt like hypocrisy that they expected us to pay sustained attention to complex material for hours. It was as if they knew better and didn't care.

In my first year, our first-quarter statistics professor wrote a mathematical proof on the chalkboard for 45 minutes. I tried to follow, catching superscripts and subscripts as best as I could. My notes were a jumbled mess, and I wanted to cry. We were halfway through class when he turned to us and said, "This isn't on the exam." I dropped my pen midair onto the page and sighed in relief. I stared blankly at the elbow pads of his tweed jacket for the rest of class.

Around that same time, I sat through an hour-long mock dissertation defense for an advanced student in our research lab. The student went on about "sensitivity" and "specificity." Everyone else in the lab nodded along. When the student finished, Dr. Burlew asked us if we had any questions. How could I have questions? I had no idea what the student had been talking about.

That's how it went, my first year. There were new words constantly.

Heuristics. Diathesis. Anxiolytic. Sublimation. Functionalism. Dissonance. Perseverate. Dysphoric. Aphasia. Catecholamine. Beneficence. Oedipus. Dyscalculia. Prosopagnosia. Xenophobia. Masochism. Operant. Triangulate.

Even words that I already knew meant something different in psychology.

Conditioning. Pilot. Adoption. Priming. Mature. Precipitating. Course. Flat. Regression. Framing. Punishment. Unconscious. Complex. Attachment. Projection. Alpha. Borderline. Positive. Exposure. Interaction. Dynamic.

And then, there were the never-ending abbreviations that everyone seemed to know except me.

APA, OPA, MPA, WPA, SEPA, ANOVA. ADHD. ASD. OCD. SUD. ECT. DT. TD. SD. DAP. TAT. CBT. WRAT. WAIS. SMI. MMPI. CFI. CI. EI. SI. HI. HTP. LP. PD. EBP. BDI. DF. EFA. GAF. GAD. SAD.

Yes, it *was* just "sad."

Like undergrad psychology classes, I was still on the edge of my seat listening to the material, except this time, I was hanging on for dear life. The workload had quintupled compared to my undergraduate studies and was dense. Study, study, study. Evenings. Weekends. Individual study. Group study. Study with the graduate TA (Teaching Assistant).

The statistics TA was ahead of us in the program by a year or two. He was reviewing a sample analysis on a handheld whiteboard.

"One caveat you have to consider is …"

I raised my hand. He pointed to me.

"What's a 'caveat'?" I asked, thinking it was a new, unfamiliar statistical term.

A white man in my cohort turned toward me. "You don't know what *that* means?" he raged audaciously.

"No!?" I retorted, my eyes silently questioning whether he had a problem with that.

The TA broke the tension, explaining that caveat meant "warning" and resumed the lesson. I was humiliated. I didn't know psychology or English words ostensibly. I didn't belong. I was an impostor.

I first learned about the impostor phenomenon (IP) among Black students[2] during a professional development series at Dr. Burlew's research lab meeting. IP is a pervasive psychological pattern of inadequacy, self-doubt, and the persistent fear of being exposed as a "fraud" despite high achievement. It affects individuals across various backgrounds and demographics but is more common among women and racial and ethnic minorities. A poisonous cocktail of systemic racism, gender bias, and adverse childhood experiences (ACEs) placed this unrelenting pressure on me to excel in the face of adversity, but no matter what I attained, I felt like a phony. There was a name for this feeling; other people felt it, too. I wasn't alone. I wasn't fooling people. I was finding myself, my voice.

**

"Women are dumber in math," my *developmental psychology* professor lectured as I sat in the front row. I looked up from my notebook in disbelief. This must be a joke. He leaned back in his chair with his legs crossed and continued musing. I looked around at my classmates; no one else seemed to have flinched. Their heads were down, waiting to jot down the next key point from his exposition. My hand shot up in the air. The middle-aged man called on me.

"I'm sorry. Did you say, 'Women are *dumber* in math'?"

"Yes. Studies show that men outperform women on certain mathematical tasks and …"

I interrupted. I was usually 100% respectful to my elders and especially my instructors. Still, by my second year of graduate school, I was over casual sexism, racism, and classism being presented as facts.

"I can't argue against research, but I'm sure those researchers did not publish a paper that said 'women are dumber.'"

Pens froze, and the whole class turned and looked at me.

"Uh, well, yes, you're right. It didn't say that," the professor stammered before continuing his pontifications on human learning.

**

In graduate school, it was as if the high school nerds were now the bullies. Intellect was the new flex. People used the prestige and power of the professorate to push others around, especially lowly students. The administrators would say that graduate programs had more "flexibility" than on the undergraduate level. Flexible meant that the class could be four hours even though you only got three credits. Our classes ended when the professor was good and ready to stop and not a moment sooner. If a weekday class fell on a national holiday, we were expected to come in on the weekend. Research labs and clinical practicums didn't observe holiday, spring, or summer breaks. If a professor gave you and another student a racially laced nickname such as "The Golden Twins," you said nothing. You took it if another professor yelled at you, the TA, for not starting her class when she was late. When a professor assigned 96 statistics pages to read in two days, you did it. "Suggested" readings were on the exam. If a professor informed you that you would fail their class before it started, you did.

**

"You should drop my class and take a remedial course," my second statistics professor, Chuck, advised after I failed his Winter pretest.

We'd been given a booklet to study over the holidays, our first year of graduate school. Two-thirds of the questions on the exam didn't come from the reading. I blanked on math I hadn't used since the 8th grade and missed a question on negative exponents. I'd never learned to do matrices that were on the exam, and the booklet he'd given us had been of no help. To me, the test was not a fair assessment of my abilities. Please give me the right things to study or teach me the material, and then test me before issuing a verdict. I didn't drop the class. He didn't like it. I passed.

That is, I passed the first of Chuck's two courses. It wasn't over. During the Spring quarter, he seemed more motivated to prove himself right. He also appeared to be on some downward spiral. He'd lost about 30 lb but continued wearing his ill-fitting clothes. He seemed to have combed his hair with his fingers. His eyes were wide and red. He was always sweaty despite sitting still. His mood went from bad to worse.

Chuck had been the beloved statistics professor from "The Golden State.". Everyone raved about him. In three years he'd gotten tenure early and secured his position as the "golden child" of the department. When I interviewed for admissions, he'd offered, "I look forward to seeing you this Fall." It meant a lot to me for a long while.

One year later, Chuck spent the first third of class telling us we were "stupid" in different iterations. He mostly talked to his computer monitor facing the window, almost like we weren't there. His words were emotionally abusive.

"Do you know that the average IQ of students at the university, where I attended, is 10 points higher than students at the University of Cincinnati?"

How did he know this? Who would've studied it? It sounded like a fake statistic. I now knew that was a thing.

"I bet you don't even know why there's a hole in Lifesavers candy. It's so that if you accidentally swallow it, you won't choke."

Myth.

"Some of you are the same age as me, but did you know that I am the youngest person to get tenure in the history of this department."

"Did you know that there is a correlation between your admissions GRE quant scores and your performance on my midterm? Study this chart I made."

Chuck posted a regression analysis, a statistical procedure used to make predictions of our test and GRE scores on the overhead projector. There were no names, but it was easy to figure out as our cohort was small. He'd bragged about students he'd recruited with exceptional GRE scores. That's two. One person told me about her GRE scores—another one. Several had shared their test scores—four more. I knew mine. One. At least eight of us were outed in an instant.

We complained to the Chair that it was a FERPA violation of our privacy. Chuck's defense was that he had "deidentified" the data. He was told not to do it again, but getting called out didn't stop him.

No one in the class understood Chuck's scoring methodology. I got something like a 26.97 on the Spring quarter midterm and failed, but a score of 27.01 passed. It was as if he'd deliberately set the cut point to ensure my demise. With him, it was one big shell game. To add insult to injury, my classmate, who scored 27.01, offered to tutor me. My eyebrow raised at the gesture, but I bit my tongue. However misguided and insulting it felt, I knew she meant well.

I approached Chuck after class to see what I could do about my grade. My scores on the homework assignments had been strong. The TA graded those and did not identify any lag in comprehension.

"You got the lowest grade in the class. Like I told you before, you need some remediation in an undergraduate course."

"Oh no, that wasn't me. I got the grade just below the cutoff mark for passing," I said, feeling pleased and expecting my chances for assistance were now better.

Chuck's eyes widened, but he quickly reverted to his original destination.

"Well, there's still no way for you to pass my class. There's always a strong correlation between performance on my midterm and finals. It's statistically impossible. You will fail."

We had a significant homework assignment due the following week. Chuck told us that under no circumstances were we to work together. I skipped our usual study group and dredged through the assignment independently. I turned it in on the due date, anxious about what I'd done alone until classmates reassured me that they'd taken the same steps.

We were hardly seated for the next class before Chuck started in. His face was red, and spittle projected onto his computer monitor occasionally.

"I told you all NOT to work together. Some of you did anyway and that's cheating. This is a violation of the Graduate Student Handbook. I will prosecute you to the fullest extent possible. I could have you kicked out of graduate school," he threatened.

He rambled on for like 84 minutes. I half listened. I'd learned to tune out his tantrums to keep him from getting in my head. It was an emotional escape. His tirade also didn't apply to me, so I felt free to ignore him. Chuck was so furious that he ended class early. He wanted us out of his sight.

Relieved at our early release, I gingerly began packing up my belongings. Then, Chuck continued.

"All of you can leave, but Bridgette and Cara, I need you to stay behind."

I froze mid-air with my stats notebook hovering over the designated slot in my shoulder bag. I looked up over my computer monitor as the blood drained from the upper portions of my body. Expressions of concern, shock, and relief passed across my classmates' faces as they hurried to exit the computer lab. Cara and I passed a wide-eyed glance at each other, momentarily unsure what the other might have done during our temporary separation.

We were the only two Black people in our cohort. We were from the same research lab, had all our classes together, and sometimes went to the same church, yet we were completely different.

Cara had lived a sheltered life, and I had not. I sometimes resented feeling like a surrogate mother helping her navigate adulthood, though I was grateful that we were academic partners. Years later, I found out she shared similar sentiments toward me, both grateful and resentful. Ultimately, we'd agreed that we were great colleagues but fell short of friends. Allies in the war against Chuck though, we made our way to the front of the room, braced for the next battle.

Chuck's eyes were now relaxed, and his posture was open. I pushed down the knot in my throat, tears and bile begging for release. Cara tugged at the sagging knees of her size 0 jeans.

"So, I wanted to see how you all were coping with the riots and everything happening in the city?"

My adrenaline was pumping, not downshifting to relief at the unexpected topic. Was he serious? Didn't he know what message he had just sent to the class? Did he realize how much stress he'd caused for us?

Cara recovered first.

"I'm doing okay. It's hard to watch what's happening, but I'm staying busy with school."

Her response gave me enough time to quiet the clapbacks I'd formulated that yearned to call Chuck everything but a child of God.

"Yeah, me too."

Three words was all I could muster. I avoided his probing blue eyes. He would've seen the truth in my raised eyebrow. I was still working on my clinical poker face. The one where a patient says something shocking and you can keep it together. My first clinical supervisor would say, "Bridgette, it's all over your face," as she observed my early therapy sessions. I tried to relax my face as Chuck feigned racial allyship and blabbered some words intended to be comforting before releasing us from his vice grip.

***

One night at the end of my first year, I paced the long hallway of my first apartment, waiting for my stats grades to come out. I'd studied all night and all day between and after classes for 10 days. I hadn't gotten a whole night's sleep or eaten a real meal in that time. My blue book was bursting with excessive explanations of each concept on the exam to ensure that I was clear. I had never worked so hard at school in my entire life.

Grades are so automatized now that I cannot recall how the news came. I can only remember my reaction.

"C+" was the call. I'd failed. It was the first time that hard work didn't work. It was a novel feeling for me. Rather than standing as a single point, one grade, one moment, I let it define me. I was a failure.

I flung myself across my bed and had one of those sobbing until your stomach cramps type of cries. I hugged my knees to my chest to ease the pain. My comforter darkened with tears, saliva, and snot. I didn't care. I was broken.

Through blurry, wet eyes, I saw a yellow plastic shopping bag next to my face on the bed. I moved to shove it to the floor to make room for my continued grieving, but something caught my eye. I'd never noticed it before. The black print on the bottom of the bag read "John 3:16."

The bag was from Forever 21, a fashion clothing retailer for young adult women. I'd shopped at the store many times, but I'd never seen the Bible verse on the bag before that moment. Granny had drilled us with memory verses we recited each quarter in front of the church. I knew it by heart.

"For God so loved the world, that he gave his only begotten Son, that whosoever believeth in him should not perish, but have everlasting life."

It was like a sobering splash of icy water. It was a reassurance to me that there was something bigger in control. Religion had given me a foundation, a feeling of safety and security in my childhood. I sat up on the bed and wiped my face with both hands. I didn't know what would happen but knew I'd be alright. It took me a year to find out.

On the one hand, sitting in a statistics class of first-year graduate students as a second-year student was embarrassing. On the other hand, I'd already passed the following two advanced statistics courses in the sequence with As under a different instructor and rebuilt some confidence. I was doing well on my clinical rotations. I'd gotten one of the highest grades in what was alleged to be the most challenging course in our training, *Sensation and Perception,* which deals with how we detect, organize, and interpret sensory information in our environment. A classmate asked me for help after failing the midterm for that class. I'd assumed everyone had passed since I'd done so well. I was wrong. My classmate's request helped me to realize that we all had different strengths and weaknesses. My cohort would go on to leverage that awareness to make our way through the program together.

Chuck continued criticizing the new 1st-year cohort as I sat with them as far back as possible. I could finish his insults in tandem and mostly tuned him out. But, as he'd prophesied, I failed his midterm. Once again, it was right below the point of passing. This time, it was no surprise, so I was less emotional. I'd suspected he was out to get me before, but now it seemed straightforward. There was no way that I hadn't comprehended the repetitive material for a second time. I went to his office hours after class to find a solution.

I knocked on Chuck's open office door. He jumped and stuffed the papers back into his briefcase. He was too late. I'd already seen that he'd been reading the "anonymous" mid-quarter course evaluations we'd just submitted in his class. We'd always been encouraged to be honest and not to fear retaliation, but now I knew for sure. He was biased and unethical.

I pretended as if I hadn't seen what he was doing. I pleaded with his ego and asked him to help me figure out where I'd gone wrong on the exam.

"You understand the material. You don't write it the way I want," he concluded.

That didn't make sense to me. Understanding seemed to be the entire point of learning. Chuck and I went in verbal circles as I stood in the doorway, never invited to sit. I asked for examples of appropriate responses, tutoring, some mercy, and anything that would keep me from failing again and getting kicked out of school. Finally, he offered a solution.

The following week, Chuck sent a scathing email to the class and cc'd the department chair and the rest of the department leadership. It read, "Since some of you would rather take a bypass than do the work, I am giving you all As. You will still be required to attend class and turn in your homework for the last two weeks of the quarter."

Pure joy washed over me when I read the significant parts of his three-paragraph rant. It was finished. It sounded as if something serious had happened. I didn't know what, and I didn't care. I was busy doing an elaborate happy dance.

The next day, to my utter disbelief, I found out that all of the commotion was about me. Chuck's proposed solution had been for my matriculation committee to vote for me to bypass his class since I'd gotten As in four other statistics classes. This is not something that I would have ever thought to do since I hardly understood the graduate academic system. However, after my committee approved it, Chuck claimed to know nothing about it.

My perception of reality had never been questioned with such intensity outside of my experiences with my mother. The difference was now I had a name for it: gaslighting. I was learning a lot in a tremendously short time. Gaslighting is a subtle type of emotional abuse used to create a false narrative. It can be so intense that it makes you second-guess your perceptions and memories.[3] The impact is exponentially more substantial when there are power differences, as with parents or teachers. Even though I had a label for the act and understood it from a personal and clinical perspective, I hadn't yet developed alternative tools to deal with it. I reverted to my usual reaction and prepared to defend my honor.

I requested an emergency meeting with the Department Chair, Dr. Corcoran. I sat nervously across from his desk, ready to clear my name. When the Chair realized what the meeting was about, he gently but abruptly stopped me.

"I am fully aware of Chuck's antics and am already working on a plan to address it."

My back softened a little in my seat. This was not how I expected this to go. I usually had to convince people, my family, and others, that my mother had altered or generated a new reality. I'd point out gaps, enlist corroborating witnesses, and sometimes state the obvious, like, "I wasn't even there when that happened."

The Chair had taken all of the wind out of my argument. He believed me. As a clinical psychologist, he took it a step further and alluded to a probable cause.

"You know about substance use from my class and your research lab, right? You also learned about personality disorders. Think about that."

My mouth clamped shut as the puzzle pieces conjoined seamlessly. It explained everything. The sudden change in appearance. The erratic behavior. The attacks. The lies. I left the Chair's office walking easy. Knowing I wasn't the problem was a significant step to recovering from two years of emotional abuse with Chuck.

The following week, Chuck spent the entirety of our last class shooting blanks in my direction and missing every time. I daydreamed about graduation. I doodled in my notebook. I counted the tiles on the ceiling. I'd been through this battle before. I knew the moves. It was the last stand in a long war. He lost.

I survived, but my self-esteem was battered and bruised. Fortunately, I had tools for healing at my disposal. Sharing my story and listening to other students with similar challenges helped me process the experience.[4] I continued to focus on the things that were within my control. I established a reasonable study routine. I prioritized sleep. I took an introspective assessment of my strengths and put my focus there. I set boundaries and limits with others despite their perceived status. I was hungry for success. In time, the abuse I experienced became less and less central to my life until, one day, I looked up, and it was gone. I completely forgot.

I never planned to go into academia and become a professor. That first lecture told me that I'd never be a good teacher. That statistics class suggested that I could never be a researcher. My first supervisor said I would be a "decent" clinician. Almost no one expected me to be here. I was an educator professor, assistant professor, and associate professor with tenure, moved and was an associate professor without and then with tenure again. In all, I earned the final rank of full professor 20 years after my first week in graduate school.

My old friend and classmate, Dr. Candace Johnson, texted me, "Congratulations." She added, "If Chuck could see you now."

I paused with zero recollection.

"Chuck who?"

References

1. Clance, P. R., & Imes, S. A. (1978). The impostor phenomenon in high achieving women: Dynamics and therapeutic interventions. *Psychotherapy: Theory Research and Practice, 15*, 241–247.
2. Ewing, K. M., Richardson, T. Q., James-Myers, L., & Russell, R. K. (1996). The relationship between racial identity attitudes, worldview, and African American graduate students' experience of the imposter phenomenon. *Journal of Black Psychology, 22*(1), 53–66.
3. American Psychological Association (APA). (2023). *Gaslight. APA dictionary of psychology.* https://dictionary.apa.org/gaslight
4. Gillihan, S. (2019, March 6). *The healing power of yelling your trauma story. Psychology Today.* https://www.psychologytoday.com/us/blog/think-act-be/201903/the-healing-power-telling-your-trauma-story#:~:text=The%20biggest%20benefit%20from%20sharing,finding%20a%20sense%20of%20meaning.%22

CHAPTER 11

Rules Are Made to Be Broken … or Bent

<u>Naming Adverse Childhood Experiences</u>

Acknowledging and naming the abuse tied to ACEs can be a transformative step in healing. The act of labeling the trauma brings clarity and validation, allowing survivors to move beyond the shame, confusion, and denial that can surround childhood abuse.[1]

"I LOVE YOU."

Damien towered above me, holding me tight and staring lovingly into my eyes. His silver-rimmed glasses slid down his nose. The center of his plaid dress shirt smelled of Polo cologne, familiar and strange at the same time.

My insides froze. We'd only been dating for a month. Four weeks. Thirty days. We hadn't even reached the end of a 90-day trial. It was too soon, for me, at least.

Damien maintained his gaze, dark eyes peering through my soul. I broke his stare, afraid of what he might see in there. The truth of everything I'd been through. The broken parts of me struggling to heal. It was too much pain for any one person to bear. Most people shut down when they heard too much of my story. With him, it was as if he saw me, and he didn't care. He was dead serious. He loved me. I shook the idea away. Too soon. That's the rule. "Love" wasn't going to derail my plans for school. I had things to do. Focus.

I carefully considered each potential response, the words that would preserve his ego but keep me honest.

I love you, too. Lie.

I don't love you. Harsh.

Thank you. Weird, but better than the alternatives.

"Uhhhhh, thank you." Through one eye, I peeked up at him, squinting to see how it had landed.

(dis)Honor Thy Mother: Daughterhood, Dysfunction and Deliverance, First Edition. Bridgette Peteet.
© 2026 John Wiley & Sons, Inc. Published 2026 by John Wiley & Sons, Inc.

Damien stepped back from the embrace, holding me at arm's distance. He turned his head upward and let out a deep chuckle. "Okay." He seemed to accept my response, growing accustomed to my walls of self-protection. I needed to know him on a deeper level, to test him. Literally.

Poor Damien. He was my guinea pig throughout graduate school. My first patient, if you will. Life and time are the test for most couples. I had actual tests. After a full day in the IT department at the Cincinnati Chamber of Commerce, he'd sit across from me at my kitchen table and answer questions from every practice psychological evaluation, cognitive assessment, and personality test I was learning. My initial and unofficial diagnosis? Sane and smart. He was off to a good start. Next.

Social, behavioral, and personality theories that drive human behavior needed to be considered. These theories help psychologists to understand behaviors and events and to predict patterns.

How did Damien communicate?
How did he cope with stress?
What was his relationship like with his friends? His family?

This is where I began to have concerns. During our first summer together, Damien and I got into a huge fight. He'd promised to pick up his friend from the nearby airport but needed me to drive him since he'd just had oral surgery on his wisdom teeth. No problem. I was finishing the last five minutes of a television program, but Damien wanted to leave immediately. The airport was so close that I wasn't taking the departure time seriously. Eventually growing frustrated with my delay, Damien picked up his office computer chair and slammed it back down in place.

In my mind, we broke up as soon as the chair landed right side up. I looked at him and said nothing. I grabbed my car keys and took him to get his friend in silence. I wasn't the silent treatment if I had nothing to say. I dropped them off at his house and went home to my apartment. I was done.

My tolerance for aggression and violence was zero, period. My resolve shocked Damien. He called and begged to talk about it. He stopped by and asked to speak. I eventually relented. We could at least have a conversation.

In Damien's mind, his action didn't count as violent because he hadn't done anything directly to me. For me, the line was clear and non-negotiable. Anything resembling direct or indirect verbal or nonverbal aggression was unacceptable. I recall a patient asking me years later, "What do you do when your husband calls you a b!t(h?" I regained my composure before responding, "I'm curious about what boundaries you have established in your relationship?" I wanted to say, "I wish he would!"

Nondirect aggression can be an early sign of things to come. We cannot ignore and minimize this type of behavior. We must confront it and set our expectations. Damien knew I was serious. He wouldn't get three strikes, but a second chance. We moved forward without further incident.

Damien's interpersonal relationships also gave me pause. They say you can judge a man by his friends, but one of his two friends was immature, and the other was a player. It wasn't looking good. Damien was also an only child. I worried that the stereotypes were true. They were. I'm kidding. Half kidding. Having been relatively independent since I was 15, at 22, he seemed spoiled to me. He was a grown man at the start of his career, and his mom regularly sent him clothes and care packages with his favorite childhood foods. I didn't know whether that was normal in regular families. Maybe I was being too harsh. I put a pin in these concerns and watched to see how it would weigh.

My final reservation was whether or not Damien understood and could handle the five-year sacrifice I was making for my future in graduate school. It meant long-term unemployment. "You mean you don't have a job?" Damien had asked this incredulously on our first date. It had been a blind date on my 23rd birthday, and his reaction blindsided me. Most people were usually impressed that I was in a Ph.D. program, but in his evaluation,

Damien was alarmed that I didn't work in the traditional sense. We could relate to being a full-time student and part-time employee, but that was undergrad. This was different. I needed him to understand. I was doing work, only it was academic. It was also personal. Everything I was learning, I also applied to myself. I wanted to be psychologically healthy.

***

Psychopathology and *Intervention*, two 3-hour block classes, met irregularly throughout the season at the mercy of our professor's summer travel schedule. There were about ten students in my clinical cohort that year, 70% women and 20% minority, meaning I had one other Black classmate. We were "special" because most cohorts had only one. We were also unique because we'd bonded in the trenches of *Statistics* with Chuck that Spring Quarter. I'd been the only casualty.

Still licking my wounds as we moved into the Summer Quarter, the fear of failure loomed in my mind. A second grade of C+, and I'd be kicked out of graduate school. In my mind, life would be over.Our Department Chair, Dr. Corcoran, a petite, mustached man, led our summer classes. I worried that he might hold a bias against me.

Had he heard what happened?
Was he aware that I'd failed?
Did he blame me and not the beloved Chuck?

Dr. Corcoran's class was a full year before I'd retake *Statistics* with Chuck and finally report him. I had no idea what Dr. Corcoran was thinking before that revelatory meeting a year later.

From the start, I realized that I'd stressed for nothing. Dr. Corcoran was a master educator, inspiring and training us to identify, diagnose, and treat psychological disorders with great empathy and encouragement. He had us envision gathering our treatment tools in a "bag of tricks," knowledge and skills growing exponentially in just a few months. He restored my passion for psychology and renewed my sense of self-efficacy. Once blocked by anxiety, new constructs and ideas flowed more freely through my brain, my prefrontal cortex, to be more specific.

Dr. Corcoran's class named and enhanced much of what I'd already learned in life about human behavior. I could catch subtle emotions, the microexpressions that crossed someone's face before a more acceptable facade took their place.[2,3] Since childhood, I was attuned to what people said, watched what they did, and noticed the difference between them. In class, I learned that observation is a therapist's greatest tool. It wasn't just about what words people said, but what they equally left out. Maybe, more importantly, it was about behavior. The discord between someone's words and emotions or their beliefs and actions tells the more accurate truth.

As a child, I couldn't understand my ability to anticipate seemingly predictable outcomes while grownups often forged ahead as if blind to the probable consequences. I'd been ear-hustling in adult conversations since I was five years old. The secret was to stay silent and not ask questions to draw attention to yourself. I figured out a lot myself and came to perceptually limited conclusions for the rest. If you don't pay your rent, you get evicted. Finding adequate employment as an adult is more difficult if you don't go to school. Having a child when you aren't ready is burdensome. If you hook up with a rotten man, he'll do evil things. The cause and effect were evident, and I was excessively judgmental when other people didn't see it. Then, education gave me a name for the human drives, defense mechanisms, cognitive distortions, and trauma responses that impair rational thinking. I better understood the desire to seek immediate pleasure despite the long-term consequences. No one is immune to the influence of our mind's attempts to protect us, but insightful people are better at sorting through the clutter and considering alternative perspectives. We, in turn, learned to help patients explore these different vantage points and make more informed decisions for their benefit.

As an undergraduate in *Abnormal Psychology*, I'd already learned about 40 or so different disorders, such as depression, anxiety, psychotic, and eating disorders. I'd read the essential characteristics of each illness and had a general sense of the major signs. I could see these symptoms in other people, especially certain family members. I waited to come across mine. Surely, I had a mental illness, too. I'd gone through too much and been blamed for so much. I never found it, but I didn't realize how little I knew. In graduate school, I learned that there was much more to diagnosing than lists.

In Dr. Corcoran's *Psychopathology* class, we used the *Diagnostic and Statistical Manual of Mental Disorders* (*DSM*) to learn about the scientific roots underlying the classifications of mental illness. We examined the etiology of psychiatric conditions, meaning the genetic and environmental contributors such as substance use or underlying medical conditions. We were trained to differentiate between disorders with similar symptoms. With "depression" there were about 10 different types, including major depressive disorder, postpartum depression, seasonal affective disorder, and more. We practiced our clinical diagnostic interview skills and, later, structured measures, each with targeted or specific lines of questioning to help assess and diagnose mental illness in hypothetical cases. We learned how to sort the relevant from the irrelevant in the information we received from our patients and move sessions along. Early in my training, I asked a patient, "How much do you drink?" She started down a long path about the failures of her water intake. I meant alcohol.

Proper diagnosing is crucial. It informs treatment selection. It affects how we provide psychoeducation to patients about their illness. It's a shorthand communication to other professionals. Plus, without a diagnosis, insurance won't usually pay for treatment.

Conversely, some psychologists argue that diagnosing is overused and can prevent people from getting the help that they need. I saw this firsthand when a friend's son was exhibiting symptoms of attention-deficit hyperactivity disorder (ADHD). I suspected that the father also had it. Since psychologists cannot treat friends and family, I gave them a referral. An accurate diagnosis requires a complex, well-rounded evaluation from an adequately trained person. ADHD is a commonly overused and abused diagnosis, and I wanted to be sure. The U.S. Food and Drug Administration (FDA), in 2023, reported an Adderall shortage due to the inability to keep up with the demand for these medications.[4] Ultimately, the boy's test results confirmed my suspicions; however, the parents declined treatment because it was stigmatizing. Careless labeling creates treatment barriers and shouldn't be done.

"Don't walk around diagnosing people who aren't your patients. It's unethical," Dr. Corcoran lectured.

At first, this was tough. I could see pathology everywhere. I knew things written off as sadness, moodiness, or attention-seeking were likely depression, bipolar, and personality disorders. It was unlikely that Uncle had extreme mood swings because someone "spiked his drink" in college. Hearing voices is not "quirky." Dementia is not a normal part of aging. Sharing what I knew without coming across as a know-it-all was becoming a tricky balance.

I saw movies in an entirely new light. Psychological thrillers that used to cause week-long bouts of insomnia lost their magic with inaccurate portrayals of mental illness. No, the movie killer doesn't have an "Axis 5 disorder." That's not a thing. I've ruined a few movies for my family by pointing out these errors. While learning about disorders, I also learned how to treat them.

In our new role as psychologists in training, we weren't giving advice like an older sibling or a good friend. We weren't relying on catchphrases to make people feel better, like "Positive Vibes Only." All emotions are okay; what you do with them can cause problems. We weren't conjuring up activities that sound good but are largely ineffective, such as punching a pillow to address anger. Inappropriate and poorly timed psychological interventions could traumatize people further, worsen their mood, or fail to defuse the risk of harm to themselves or others.

Grounded in scientific evidence, we learned various therapeutic techniques to help patients name, identify the source, and change problematic thoughts, emotions, and behavior associated with their mental illness. We considered the validity of those treatments given the context of the patient's identity, such as age, gender, and culture, and how to adapt our approach. We learned when to make referrals for complementary medication and how to provide oversight of patient adherence and the side effects of new drugs. Our interventions were much deeper than the stereotypical therapist question, "How do you feel about that?"

And then came the most essential tool, the self. Dr. Corcoran argued that we all needed to try therapy. We should ensure our optimal mental health before taking care of others. We needed to work through our issues, past or present, and understand ourselves and what made us tick. Therapy would also be vital as we began to carry the weight of our patients' confidential problems, secrets, and traumas.

Personal therapy seemed like an unusual idea for most of us. What was he trying to say? We presumed ourselves to be psychologically healthy as mental health trainees making our way through a demanding program. But Dr. Corcoran pushed us. Therapy didn't require a full-on psychological disorder to reap the benefits. I wasn't entirely sold. I thought back to the only time I'd tried therapy. It hadn't gone well.

My best friend went to the college psychological services center as an undergraduate for what we would later know to be recurring depression. We were just 20 then, and my friend seemed far more stable than me. She'd grown up middle-class with two parents who loved her. That wasn't her entire story, but I figured that if *she* was having problems, I should certainly go to therapy. I had been through a lot but was never allowed to talk about my problems uninhibitedly.

Talking, though, meant violating the code of family secrecy. The code that applied to the fun inside jokes and confidential cookie recipes, but, more importantly, to the traumatic, abusive, toxic experiences forced to remain unspoken. Therapy was my loophole. No one in my family would know. As a bonus, it was free because I was a student.

I was nervous when I called to schedule an appointment, but the intake therapist, Amy, eased my concerns with her calming voice. She asked me a few general questions about my age, gender, race, and the nature of my problem. She scheduled me for a full intake the following week.

I entered the third-floor suite, worried that someone would recognize me. I glanced at the downturned faces in the waiting room. Strangers. I was safe. After a few minutes, a door to a hallway of offices opened, and a tiny blonde woman about my age called my name. I walked toward her, noting her pale purple cardigan and khakis. Amy smiled, introduced herself, and asked me to follow her.

Safely inside the nondescript room, I sat across from Amy in a stiff office chair. She started talking first. She may have mentioned that she was in training. I hope she informed me about the limits of confidentiality as required by law, but all I remember is when it was my turn to talk, the floodgates opened. My complex history came rushing out, pushing Amy against the back of her chair. After 50 short minutes, time was up. I happily agreed to return the following week. I bounced back to my dorm, feeling slightly hopeful.

I arrived for my second session, still riding the high of hope. As soon as I sat down, I could tell something was off. Amy sat awkwardly in her chair, unsure what to do with her hands. Her eyes darted away from my questioning eyes.

Maybe she's having a lousy day. I brushed it off and sat ready to go again. I had so much to tell her.

Amy began talking, but her voice wavered, "How has your mood been over the past week?"

"I felt pretty good after we talked last time."

Her question felt like a formality, like when people ask, "How are you doing?" and they want you to say "Fine" and not give an honest answer.

Amy barely acknowledged my response as she rushed toward her true agenda.

With a gulp, she mumbled, "Something came up in your session last week."

Mentally, I sped through everything I'd shared. *I was in excellent health. There were no official mental illnesses in my immediate family, but my mom had a lot of issues. My parents were divorced, and I had four siblings. My maternal grandparents finished raising me. School was going well, and I was trying to make something out of my life.* We'd covered a lot of ground, but I hadn't told her a fraction of the craziness yet. What could she possibly be talking about?

"You told me that the last time you were home, your mother sent your little sister to get her marijuana for her."

Huh? Her statement hit me out of the blue. I was confused. Amy must be confused, too. That hadn't been the point of my story. I was sure I could fix this with a more precise explanation. She'd asked me if I used drugs, and I'd told her what happened the last time I went home.

On a recent trip to Delaware, I'd gone over to visit my mother. She now lived in a one-bedroom efficiency apartment with my adult brother, his best friend, my 8-year-old sister, and our Dad's cousin. Four adults and one child living in two rooms—troubling. Our mother dating our first cousin once removed on our Dad's side—disturbing, but that's beside the point.

We were playing Spades in the eating area. Mom called Tanya to bring her weed pipe from the bedroom. My heart sank. I hated smoke. Mom knew it. I wanted to leave, but I also wanted to fit in with my family, so I stayed. Mom lit the pipe and started smoking. My stomach turned. My brother and his friend took their hits of the purple glass pipe in turn, blowing clouds of smoke above their heads in mini deference to me. On the next round, Mom inhaled, but instead of exhaling up or out in front of her, she turned directly to her right, toward me. And blew the smoke directly into my face. It was as if she believed I'd become instantly high, relax, and not take offense. Her plan failed. Through the haze, I'm unsure if she saw misery or rage in my eyes. She offered "I forgot" in faux atonement.

"But *I* didn't smoke," I emphasized this point, hoping it would ease Amy's concerns. Recreational marijuana was illegal, and I thought this would call off the alarm.

"It's not about you smoking. It's about your sister. She's underage."

"Oh, well, she wasn't in the room while they were smoking." Amy was missing my point.

"Yes, but I talked with my supervisor, and she said that having a child handle drug paraphernalia is against the law."

Child. Law. My stomach flipped.

"I'm obligated to make a report if you are a danger to yourself or others and if children or the elderly are being abused?"

Report. It had only been five years since the last one that had turned our lives upside down. My chest tightened. My eyes filled up.

"Yeah, but 'abuse' is like physically hurting somebody."

"It's more than that. It includes child safety and well-being, too," she corrected.

I was glad I hadn't told her more about what happened to me as a child. This could've been way worse, I thought. Amy continued.

"I have the telephone number here for Child Protective Services in your hometown. We can call them together, or I can do it after our session."

There was no air in the room. I stayed, slumping in my seat. I wanted to know what Amy was going to say. I had to warn my family. I was relieved when she couldn't say much. She had my mother's and sister's first name, no address. I didn't even know it. Amy turned to me to fill in the blanks when she couldn't answer their questions, and I made no effort to help her. My mother and sister also had different last names than me and from each other. My stomach unknotted slightly. It's pretty easy to find someone in a small town. After about five minutes, Amy ended the call and resumed fidgeting.

"How are you feeling now?" she asked, finding my eyes this time.

"How do you *think* I am feeling?" I snapped, calling her every name but her own in my head. "I came to you for help with my problems, and what did you do? You gave me more! My mother is going to kill me, thanks to YOU!" I seethed. *Crap, maybe I shouldn't have said that last part. She might think my life is really in danger.*

Amy didn't respond. Instead, she started sobbing. I softened a bit. Tears have that effect on most people. I didn't yet know they could be weaponized.

"Why didn't you tell me this last week when I told you this story?" I continued, not ready to completely calm, but moving down from level 10.

"Because I'm in training and didn't know," Amy offered helplessly.

"Well, they need to train you better. You can't just blindside someone with a thing like that!"

"What do you want to do?" Amy asked between sobs, pulling tissues from the box usually reserved for the patients.

"Leave. Can I leave?"

"Yes, of course."

Feigning toughness, I stormed past Amy's chair and out the door of the office and suite. As I walked toward my dorm, my heavy steps switched to slow, tentative ones. The fear in my stomach had made its way up to my throat, gripping it like a clamp. I imagined it was my mother's large hands around my neck, draining the life out of me. She *was* going to kill me this time.

It was one of the most challenging phone calls I've ever made. My mother cut into me through the receiver. I wept as she belabored how "stupid" and "naïve" I was for sharing her "business." She didn't have a car and couldn't get to me. I was safe, for now. Summer was coming far too soon, though. I was supposed to return to my hometown. Instead, my Uncle Brian, Mom's youngest brother, and I plotted my escape to Connecticut for two months to babysit his kids. I would be eight hours away from her reach, just in case.

Back in Dr. Corcoran's class, I could reflect on my sessions with Amy from a newfound perspective. I knew that I needed therapy if I was ever to recover from the multifaceted traumas that I'd experienced as a child. With my accidental revelation to Amy, I'd barely scratched the surface of the complexities of my adverse childhood. I had to keep digging. Secrecy compounds trauma and is a dysfunctional but typical behavior in unhealthy family systems. By going to therapy, I'd broken the family's corrupt code of silence, but I was *not* the one who had broken the law.

Child abuse was much broader than what I'd conceptualized with an untrained eye back then. It included acts or failure of caregivers to act in any events that cause physical, emotional, sexual, or exploitative harm to children. But, even then, it's still essential to consider the context. Is the risk of injury or harm imminent? Does the parent's behavior fall outside of cultural norms? Are parenting classes a viable option? What resources are available to support single mothers and low-resourced families? What solutions cause the least amount of trauma for the children? What is the plan for family reunification if possible? With both reports, no one in the system considered this for my family. So, I would do it for my patients. Yes, I must make the call. I have a legal obligation. I can also report helpful information such as my patient is in therapy, they understand the issue and demonstrate remorse, they're working on behavior change, they've been connected to resources, and so forth, to help mitigate the impact of my report. It seems to go much better for them with this approach.

I gave Amy a lot more grace for her fumble now that I was a psychology trainee and making mistakes myself. She wasn't wrong; she just could have done better. I learned from her. Countless times, I'd delivered my spiel to clients about the limits of confidentiality, including harm to self or others, child or elder abuse, and court orders. Based on my negative experience, I took this information further to include examples and allowed my patients an opportunity to ask questions for clarity. Even so, I missed the mark in other ways.

***

During my graduate school training, I was working in a clinical practicum. I'd been treating a client for about two months. "Sarah" was 22 and experiencing a cultural identity crisis. She had been adopted from Indonesia as an infant by White parents. Her parents had made no effort to connect her to her biological or cultural roots, acting as if Sarah was "magically White," as she put it. In therapy, she was on a mission to explore where she came from, reclaim her identity, and educate her parents about their missteps. Sarah began making new Asian American friends on campus and shared a story about a boy she'd met.

"Yeah, he wanted to talk. So, he came to my dorm room last night. I didn't have any place for him to sit, so he sat on my bed. We were sitting there talking, and he got more and more comfortable. He took his shirt off, and I was a little uncomfortable, but he had a t-shirt underneath. He took his arm off and laid it on the bed between us. He kept talking about his day and moving closer to me. . .."

"I'm sorry, what did you say?" I interrupted her with no clinical grace. I'd been so engrossed with the details of her story and where I thought it might be going. A girl with a strange boy in a college dorm room, fill in the blank. She'd taken a hard left turn, and I'd missed the exit.

"Yeah, I thought it was weird that he took his arm off too."

Trying to connect the dots, I started asking dumb questions.

"Was he bleeding?" "Was it a prosthetic arm?" Make it make sense.

No, and no. I recalibrated, shaking off my confusion. I knew what it was. Psychosis. I needed to know more. I screened for the frequency of her visual hallucinations and the presence of other types, such as auditory. It wasn't the first time Sarah had experienced psychotic symptoms, but the first time she'd told anyone. This was serious. I was out of my depth. I paused my questioning.

"Will you wait here while I find a supervisor to work with us?"

Breathless, I ran through the center square of offices, trying to find help. I found one supervisor and blurted out what happened as we returned to my office. My supervisor took over the session with the ease of a seasoned professional. I stood watching.

My supervisor recounted what I'd told her and invited Sarah to fill in the blanks. I thought Sarah might change or redact her story to protect herself, but she didn't. She seemed to know that something wasn't right and wanted help. Then, I was thrown for another loop.

My supervisor probed, "Tell me about the burns on your wrist."

My eyes darted to the barely concealed stretches of gray lesions on Sarah's left forearm. The evidence of self-injury was as clear as day. I'd been so caught up in listening that I forgot observation. I was embarrassed but couldn't focus on my emotions. My supervisor wanted to switch places with me again. She'd told Sarah that we were concerned for her safety and that I'd be the one to walk her through voluntary or involuntary committal. On the inside, my heart was throbbing in my ears. On the outside, I was finally mastering a more stoic face. It would be my first time processing a psychiatric hold.

An hour later, the emergency medical technicians (EMTs) rolled Sarah away strapped to a stretcher. I promised to check in on her at the hospital. As I waved farewell, feelings of inadequacy rushed in. I turned and apologized to my supervisor for being so careless in missing the burns. She countered my self-criticism and reminded me of everything I'd done right. In the end, the patient was safe. I was in training, and mistakes were inevitable. I had to stop judging myself and others so harshly.

***

I was prepared the next time I went to therapy in my late 20s. I knew what to look for and what to expect. I found an older Black woman to work with, figuring I could skip explaining some cultural nuances unique to Black families. She helped me to process my mother's issues. I had to stop doubting myself. I was not the problem, no matter how often I'd been told otherwise. I learned to view my mother's pathology from an outside perspective. I didn't have to sit under it as a victim. I was reminded that I now knew better. I knew mental illness, the signs and symptoms. I could name what my mother had. I was familiar with the tools of psychological manipulation. I also knew the prognosis or expected outcome. There was nothing I could do to help my mother.

She would forever be the same. I had to stop fixating on her. I had to focus on myself. She wasn't the one in therapy; I was. That's usually how it goes, the victim is the one in treatment.

Through therapy, I began to see the overt and hidden ways my childhood negatively shaped my behaviors and beliefs. There were many of them—some things I'd accepted unknowingly as a part of my identity. I was the "smart sister" and not the attractive one. I was "sensitive" and couldn't take negative feedback. I was "lazy" because I wasn't a morning person, never have been. I believed I wouldn't be a decent cook because I'd once boiled a pot of water to nothing. Mom never let me live it down. My identity was rooted in what Mom said I was and what I accepted.

Sometimes, people teach us who we do not want to be. Much of the early plan for my life was to do the opposite of Mom. Stay in school. Say no to drugs. Go to church. Consider the emotions of others. Watch out for men. In therapy, I learned that there were a few flaws in my plan. I couldn't just do the reverse of my mother and find emotional health.

In my early twenties, a peculiar pattern emerged: my mother mimicked many of my actions and decisions and attempted to overshadow them. For instance, when I was admitted to grad school, Debra announced her pursuit of a "degree" in medical billing. At 23, I was baptized in the Seventh-Day Adventist Church, and shortly afterward, my mother decided to undergo a rebaptism herself. When I became engaged, she followed suit, getting engaged shortly after. The trend continued; I mentioned our consideration of moving to Arizona, and my mother spoke of having a house "on hold" there for the next eight years. Even mundane things such as switching to soy milk, learning to crochet, or scrapbooking wasn't immune to this pattern, as my mother followed in kind and became temporarily obsessed with my latest hobby. They say that imitation is the highest form of flattery, but I did not take it as a compliment. It felt like my identity was being blurred, and I struggled to maintain a sense of individuality.

Basing my life on my mother in any way, opposite or not, left me without an independent identity. Who was I separate from her and her influence? I had to figure it out. It started with burning the original script I'd created for my life. It had gotten me pretty far, but it was time for a new chapter. It took about five years, in my early 20s, to write it. The first year, I opened up to accept healthy love.

***

It was Thanksgiving of 2001, six months after I'd first met Damien. We'd gone our separate ways for the holiday, him back to Detroit and me back to Delaware. I remember feeling down that we weren't together to celebrate. It didn't feel right. We'd been through a lot in that short time. He'd helped me through failing my first-year statistics class. I'd nursed him through his wisdom teeth extraction. He'd rushed to my side when neighbors were fighting and helped me move when I had a Peeping Tom. That first September, we'd sat together watching the attacks on the World Trade Center at a loss for words. My family had met him several times and had fallen in love with him, but I was holding out.

My sister, Devon, and I processed all of this as we sat on the floor of our old bedroom at Granny and Pawpaw's house. We hadn't seen many successful relationships growing up. It was tricky to judge what was normal or healthy. Devon understood my hesitancy, the fear of failure, and the price of making the wrong decision. But, with just a few words, she broke down my walls.

"You know it's okay to like him."

And so, I did. Damien and I were engaged a year later.

All the while, I continued working to dismantle my self-beliefs and create a new identity in the following years. I didn't have to prove myself in school to earn my mother's approval. I would never get it. Education became a tool for me. It helped me grow in countless ways and changed the financial trajectory of my life. Abstaining from drugs was no longer driven by a desire to be different from my mother. I understood the slippery slope that led some patients to unintentional addiction and wanted to avoid it. My views on religion evolved. I didn't accept faith without question or out of guilt. I asked questions of faith leaders and learned more about God's love rather than His wrath. Though I kept my faith, I rejected things within religious institutions that put people in harm's way, such as minimizing child abuse and marginalizing women and sexual minorities. I was finding myself.

I could be intelligent and care about my appearance, so at age 30, I took an introductory make-up application course and began experimenting. At 35, I learned to love the hair labeled "difficult" and figured out the best way to maintain my thick mane without chemicals. I worked to be less responsive to negative feedback. For example, I do not let one critical comment in a course evaluation ruin my week. I stopped thinking of my sleep habits as "lazy." Sleep is essential to mental and physical health; some people need more sleep than do others to function optimally. I was one of them. To learn to cook, I sat at Granny's kitchen counter throughout my 20s and observed. She'd smack my hand away when I tried to capture and measure a "smidge," "pinch," or "heap" of some ingredient on a spoon or in a cup so I could write it down exactly. I got a lot better in the kitchen and life.

In my trauma response, I used to be a perfectionist, a clean freak, and an overcompensating parent. I'm slowly lessening the pressure. Control is a difficult thing for me and others who have experienced trauma to release. I grew up in chaos, and control gave me a sense of stability, order, and safety. A bit of control is positive and healthy, but like with most things, there can be too much. I eventually learned that I couldn't control everything. When you're married, your partner's choices also affect you. Children need space to grow and learn from their mistakes without excessive restrictions. And life will happen to everyone no matter how much you plan. No one is exempt from difficulty, tragedy, sickness, or death touching their lives. I had to work in a part of me that could go with the flow at times, accept that chaos would come, and find comfort with the unknown.

Despite all the work I've put in to recover from my adverse childhood experiences (ACEs), I still stumble across remnants of unhealed wounds that affect my identity. Recently, I made a new friend. I try not to take myself too seriously and joke a lot. My new comrade laughed at my antics and often said how witty I was. Amidst our giggles, I'd tell her, "Wait until you meet my sister, Devon; she's so much funnier than me." I'd apparently stated this to her several times until she pointed it out one day. She wondered why I always minimized my humorous qualities.

In 40 years, I'd never thought about being funny. I was stunned. I reflected on it. The remnants of our "boxes." The thing that said who each child was in Mom's estimation. I reframed my thinking again. Devon and I could both be amusing; it was allowed. We could be our whole selves irrespective of the other person. We weren't reduced to one. We weren't in competition. We weren't limited to what others said, what Mom said. I was becoming me.

References

1. Psychology Today. (n.d.). *Parental abuse.* https://www.psychologytoday.com/us/basics/parenting/parental-abuse
2. Porter, S., & ten Brinke, L. (2008). Reading between the lies: Identifying concealed and falsified emotions in universal facial expressions. *Psychological Science, 19,* 508–514.
3. Vrij, A., Granhag, P. A., & Porter, S. (2010). Pitfalls and opportunities in nonverbal and verbal lie detection. *Psychological Science in the Public Interest, 11*(3), 89–121. https://doi.org/10.1177/1529100610390861
4. U.S. Food and Drug Administration (FDA). (2023). *FDA announces shortage of adderall.* https://www.fda.gov/drugs/drug-safety-and-availability/fda-announces-shortage-of-adderall

CHAPTER 12

The Verdict

Adverse Childhood Experience—Household Mental Illness

Parental mental illness is an ACE if the child was aware of the parent's mental illness and it was not effectively managed, interrupted the child's emotional and mental development, or had serious consequences for the child's development and health.[1]

INSIDE MY CHEST, my heart clenched just a little. The results were in 9-8. As faulty, we'd never had a split decision like this. We liked to be unanimous, on one accord, like a jury. At most, one person might abstain while the rest stayed in sync. This time, we were fully divided, nearly in half. Those in favor of remediation for the student had won. Those of us for dismissal weren't convinced change was possible. Neither group rested easy.

I hung the white flag of surrender. It was the best I could hope for in this scenario. She, the student, hadn't been able to sway almost half of us, a mini victory in a fight that usually favored the master manipulator. Her win might've been impressive if it weren't so scary. A room of 17 clinical psychology professors, and 9 of them had fallen for the Siren's song. Some of us had traversed this path many times before and were all too familiar with that dangerous tune.

"Thank you for coming in today, Ashley. We're here to discuss the recent accusation of plagiarism in Dr. Peteet's Cultural Diversity class." The Dean of Students led the panel along with two other faculty.

Ashley, a psychology doctoral student, was dressed to the nines in a business suit with her blonde hair slicked back into a tight bun. It was as if she couldn't help batting her long eyelashes at you when she spoke. She'd entered the conference room, portfolio in hand, ready to defend her case as if she were in a court of law. And defend she did.

(dis)Honor Thy Mother: Daughterhood, Dysfunction and Deliverance, First Edition. Bridgette Peteet.
© 2026 John Wiley & Sons, Inc. Published 2026 by John Wiley & Sons, Inc.

"I'm offended that Dr. Peteet would make such an accusation. In all my years of school, nothing like this has ever come up. I'm attending an Ivy next year. Why would I risk that? Perhaps Dr. Peteet is confused, and I can clarify."

Ashley held a disarming smile and cool-kid confidence that bordered on cocky. She wasn't actually "attending" an Ivy League; she'd be working at an institution for her clinical internship year with children no less, but name-dropping added a shroud of credibility. She'd also attempted to downgrade the issue to a misunderstanding and deflect responsibility to me.

Typical consequences for plagiarism include earning a zero on the assignment, automatically failing the course, academic probation, or expulsion. This varies by institution and severity of the offense. Traditionally, the bar is higher in terminal degree programs. At the doctoral level, we see ourselves as gatekeepers of the psychology profession and commit to abiding by and enforcing a stringent code of ethics. We must protect the public from potential harm at the hands of our trainees.

"Here is a copy of the Social Identity Life Map you submitted for your assignment. Here is a printout of the same one found on the internet. We'd like to hear what you have to say?"

"Well, Dr. Peteet didn't give clear instructions for the assignment," Ashley evaded.

One of the faculty members slid a third piece of paper across the conference room table toward Ashley. "Dr. Peteet provided us a copy of the guidelines provided. It's six bullet points written in red font."

"But, she didn't say it had to be 'original,' " Ashley sat back in her seat, confident in her deflection.

" 'Original' is written here in all caps in her instructions," another faculty member pointed at the page.

"This is graduate school, and you should've known long before now that ALL assignments have to be original," the first faculty member retorted.

Ashley pivoted, "Actually if you look closely, my assignment isn't the same. I spent hours moving the timelines around. I put a lot of effort into it. That's work, and it was just one homework assignment."

"Those 'hours' could've been used to create an original assignment," the Dean of Students pointed out.

Silence.

"So, I can copy an article off the internet and change the font color, and it's not plagiarism," one faculty member asked sarcastically.

"No," Ashley responded.

"This is psychology, not a graphic design program," the other faculty member concluded.

Backed into a corner, Ashley rerouted. She dropped her face into her hands and started to sob. "Things are so hard right now. I'm busy balancing classes and practicum. Sometimes I feel overwhelmed. I respect you all so much as faculty. I hate that I disappointed you all. I don't want you to think poorly of me. Please."

The full faculty were later given a summary of the meeting. Since it was the first time Ashley had been caught cheating, the jury voted to give her an academic warning. I gave Ashley a zero on the assignment; however, its weight meant she couldn't get an "A" in my class no matter what she did. She'd have to ace the remaining assignments to avoid getting a "C," a failing grade in graduate school. Two substandard grades were grounds for dismissal. I was somewhat satisfied with the consequences. Ashley was not. She sent me a message through the online assignment portal the following week.

"I believe I *deserve* at least partial credit on this assignment because of the time I spent on it."

My ears burned at Ashley's entitlement. What'd happened to the emotional woman who didn't want to "look bad" in front of the faculty? I was instantly triggered. Different faces for different folks. I firmly believe that when people show you who they are, believe them. I saw her. I couldn't unsee it.

"It's within my purview to fail you on the assignment or the entire course. I suggest you take this zero with gratitude," I responded to Ashley with finality.

Six months later, I was gearing up for a busy spring semester. I'd survived the first day of classes and headed into a long day of meetings the following day. In the faculty meeting, the first order of business was to deal with a student who'd been dismissed from their internship over the holiday break. *Great, so much for easing into the term.*

Ashley. It was Ashley. She was at it again. On internship, she'd initiated a friend request and had been engaging on social media with one of her male teenage patients. She'd sent a DM (direct message) suggesting that they meet up. The patient's mother reported Ashley and provided screenshots of their private messages to the Human Resources Department.

Ashley initially denied the encounter before HR confronted her with the evidence. She'd also conveniently deleted her social media account. The internship site forced Ashley to resign. Her conduct had been an overt boundary violation and breach of ethics.

Now, she was back at our campus, and it was up to us, the faculty in Ashely's degree training program, to decide whether she could continue in school. Dismissing her meant she wouldn't get her doctorate or become a psychologist, but she could still work as a master's-level practitioner. This seemed like a reasonable consequence to me. Ashley could still have a career. She'd be able to feed herself. It felt like a healthy balance between holding her accountable and our obligation to protect the public.

The discipline panel met with her twice, hoping to see evidence of remorse or understanding of the potential impact on the patient. It never came. Ashely's defense was that nothing had "actually happened." In her view, it wasn't as if she had followed through on meeting with the teen patient.

As faculty, we toiled over the facts for six hours across three meetings and 54 emails, weighing remediation versus dismissal. Near the end of the third meeting, several faculty members revealed that Ashley had reached out to them personally to plead her case. They read the emails aloud, all of which sounded genuine to them. They were ready to forgive and give her a second (or third) chance. *Did ethical boundary violations and a cover-up count for one or two more strikes?* The emails were cringeworthy to me and a few others with clinical or lived experiences of individuals with personality disorders or a low tolerance for nonsense. It felt like a strategic character campaign targeting key individuals, perhaps perceived as softer or influential. We sat with knots in our guts as our work family was charmed and deceived by disingenuous emotions and tactics. The signs of a Cluster B narcissistic personality disorder (NPD) seemed obvious. They were clinical psychologists. Couldn't they see it, too?

Cluster B disorders are a set of personality disorders that include behaviors that are overly dramatic, excessively emotional, cause distress, and impair relationships. They include antisocial, borderline, histrionic, and narcissistic personality disorders. These disorders are clustered because individuals traditionally exhibit symptoms across multiple diagnostic categories.[2,3] Ashley seemed to lean more heavily toward narcissism.

Narcissism occurs on a spectrum, meaning we all may exhibit some of these traits at times. Perhaps writing this book is a sign of my propensity. At one end of the continuum, feeling good about yourself and having positive self-esteem is healthy. Still, at the other end, it manifests as extreme, persistent self-centeredness that damages social relationships. "Narcissist" is often a casual label applied to everyday self-centered human interactions; however, true NPD is rare. In the United States, the estimated lifetime prevalence ranges from 5% to 6%, that is, more than 20 million people. NPD is more common among men than women.

The *Diagnostic and Statistical Manual of Mental Disorders* (*DSM-5-TR*) describes NPD as a persistent sense of grandiosity, need for admiration, and lack of empathy that begins in early adulthood and occurs across a range of circumstances, as indicated by at least five of the nine following symptoms[2]:

1. An exaggerated sense of self-importance
2. Excessive fantasies about power, success, attractiveness, or achievement
3. A belief that they are unique or "special" and can only be understood by other high-status people
4. An expectation of constant praise and admiration
5. A strong sense of entitlement and unreasonable expectations to be given favors and advantages

6. Exploitative of others (e.g., takes advantage of others for their own gain)
7. Limited empathy or ability to recognize the feelings of others
8. Often envious of others or believes that others envy them
9. Arrogant, self-important behaviors or attitudes.

My mom, Debra, was likely a textbook narcissist embodying every symptom on the list. She had a knack for centering herself at every important event. Holidays, graduations, weddings, even funerals became stages for her to shine. For my three-line solo of Silver Bells at my second-grade concert, she wore a formal black dress, high heels, and her waist-length white fur coat. In a land of flannel, she chose fur. She manipulated the hostess and snuck into my senior-year cotillion formal, sitting loud and proud amongst the ticketed guests. Whether she was competing to be the best Thanksgiving host, demanding extra tickets for strangers to my graduation ceremony, or inserting herself into a family friend's obituary, she made sure she was always the star.

She exaggerated her accomplishments and promoted herself as nurse, though she was a medical assistant and hadn't worked in healthcare since she was fired from a clinic back when I was a teenager. She often recounted a story—one no one else seemed to remember—about how she could have gone to college and out of state but was forced to live at home by her parents after high school. She tells others that she went to college and would have been wildly successful if not for the caretaking needs or constant sabotage of her husbands, children, or parents.

She also found ways to compete and exploit my successes. There were annual hair-length and jean-size competitions against me that were never close yet Mom was always the self-proclaimed victor. If I earned good grades, won awards, or graduated she used these experiences as evidence of her superior parenting skills. Her childhood was somehow harder than ours with zero supporting evidence. Any vulnerability we showed—whether tears or honest expressions of pain—was dismissed as weakness or countered with one of her favorite refrains: "You don't know what real problems are." Empathy was her enemy.

And above all, she demanded unwavering respect, constantly reminding us that she was "the best mother in the world," even as her actions painted a very different picture.

Personality disorders tend to be permanent and are not amenable to change.[4, 5] There are no prescription drugs to be given, and even long-term therapy has limited effect in mitigating symptoms. Individuals with personality disorders typically do not go to therapy unless court ordered or facing external threats such as job, marriage, or family loss. If they do go to therapy, it is usually an attempt to validate their behavior or to challenge boundaries set by others. They will often succeed in charming therapist who may have little experience with these disorders outside of the classroom. In other words, the prognosis, or outlook, is bleak.

As a psychologist and human being, one of the most challenging populations for me to treat and engage with is Cluster B personality disorders. It's tempting because I've been trained socially and professionally to see the good in people and to believe in the power of humans to change. I have excellent boundaries and in my arrogance am sometimes fooled into believing I can modulate the behaviors of others. In some cases, I can. I do believe that you teach people how to treat you. There are behaviors that I am unwilling to accept without debate, which can come across as rigid. But, a narc is always going to narc.

Pathological hope is a distorted form of optimism that keeps us emotionally tethered to the narcissist, despite repeated harm. It fuels the belief that their behavior will change if we love them enough, endure long enough, or meet their impossible standards. This hope traps us in a cycle of anticipation and disappointment, as we cling to fleeting moments of kindness or promises that are rarely fulfilled. By focusing on the potential of who the narcissist could be, rather than who they consistently show themselves to be, pathological hope prevents us from recognizing the need to prioritize our own well-being and break free, even if that means leaving others behind.

Our individual roles within my family system (i.e., golden child, scapegoat, mascot)[6] dictated our opportunities for connection or conflict long into adulthood. My sister, Dev, and I leaned on each other for comfort, support, and survival, creating a lifelong solidarity. With Tony, these roles fostered resentment and competition that seem impossible to overcome. He hasn't yet realized that we were all victims and Mom won't change.

As I reflected on my childhood experiences, particularly during faculty meetings about Ashley, I found myself wondering if my history of pain was influencing my perspective. *Was I projecting my feelings toward my mother onto my student? Was I being too harsh in my judgments, clouded by my own brokenness?* Fortunately for Ashley, it wasn't solely up to me.

That divided verdict came down. Ashley would be permitted to stay in school, provided she complied with a detailed remediation plan. It was shocking but expected. Shocking that even psychologists weren't immune to the powers of persuasion. Expected because I'd been down this road innumerable times. Manipulators will always be able to convince someone. Half a group? Heck, half a country when it came to politics in 2016 and again in 2024. I digress, but there are two things I'm sure of with NPD: (1) there will be a next, and (2) someone will fall for it.

Narcissists have an arsenal of tools for emotional manipulation. They sporadically alternate between these strategies to keep you off kilter. If you are conscientious enough to learn their tools or become desensitized, they switch it up again. Upon reflection, I can just about mark each decade of my life with Mom's strategies. In my formative years, Mom used anger to elicit compliance and it shifted from there as I struggled to resist her power.

***

I was about 13 when Mom hobbled in from work one evening with her boyfriend Ricky's help. She was doubled over in pain, barely able to walk. I scanned her stark white nurse's uniform for signs of physical injury as my siblings and I rushed to her sides. Physically, she looked just fine. We helped ease her toward the living room, sat her down in the old brown reclining chair, and huddled closely at her feet. We gave her our full attention.

"I was pregnant," Mom announced just above a whisper.

My eyes widened. *Gross*, my first thought. Second, *past tense*. Mom continued.

"And I lost the baby today," she shared, straining her voice as if something had happened to her throat. "I gave birth in the toilet. It was a boy," Mom finished.

(Trigger warning. My mental image was graphic. Skip the next paragraph if needed.)

I immediately imagined a bloody, avocado-sized baby with a detached umbilical cord plunging into the shallow water of an industrial porcelain pool. The image played in my head on a loop. To this day, I can still retrieve the memory with clarity.

The story sounded familiar, though. A lifetime movie or an after-school public service announcement (PSA) about the dangers of a hidden teenage pregnancy and giving birth on the bathroom floor. Then, my shoulders relaxed. It was a triumph out of tragedy. There would be no new younger sibling for me to parent. Mom wouldn't be having Ricky's baby, tying us to him for life.

Even at 14, logical questions ticked through my mind, but I knew not to ask about everything I was thinking.

Wait, she'd said it was a boy. She would've had to be pretty far along to tell that.

How had we missed a pregnancy?

Ricky, Mom's soon-to-be third husband, sat silently, not cosigning a word she'd said. He had an odd expression on his face. There was a tight half-pucker in one corner where downturned lips should have been. Was it doubt? I tried *never* to fixate on him too long and shook it away.

Finally, I mustered the courage to ask a question. "Where did it happen?"

I stroked the ridiculously soft skin of Mom's right forearm.

"At work," she said, continuing to strain the words.

"Why didn't you go to the hospital?" It slipped out before I could stop myself.

"Because I work in a clinic!" My body stiffened at Mom's intensity, and I recoiled slightly.

Her reaction felt out of place. Something was off. Still, I wanted her to feel like I was there for her.

"Oh, I see," I mumbled awkwardly, continuing to cling to her.

But I didn't see it.

Losing a baby in a toilet seemed like a major health emergency, one too big for a family medicine outpatient clinic, but what did I know?

I took a second scan of Mom's clothes. Spotless. Her thin, white uniform dresses were notably sensitive to stains. On about a monthly basis, she'd say, "Check me," to make sure she hadn't had a menstrual accident. The uniform was one thing; maybe she had nothing else to wear, but the compression tights were another. Her shiny white tights were tremendously difficult to get on and off. She would've had to put them back on after all of that. Suspicious. She had no reason to lie to us, though. Then again, that'd never stopped her before.

Still caught up in the horror of it all, fear that they'd flushed the baby down the toilet. I couldn't help myself. I had to ask.

"Did they get the baby out?" I never found out.

"Why the f@!# are you asking so many questions?" Mom shrieked at me, jumping from the rocking chair and towering over our perches on the floor. I jumped back in case she decided to strike. She didn't. She shrugged our attentive shroud and stormed upstairs, shaking the old house with each step.

Seconds ago, she'd seemed too weak to walk or talk straight. Now, her voice was crisp, clear, and strong. Her limp had disappeared, too. Like an obedient puppy, Ricky followed behind her.

When they were out of earshot, one of my siblings quipped, "She's lying."

"Yeah, I know," I cosigned.

Pathological lying seemed like a genetic trait that afflicted several family members, including Mom. General lying refers to occasional or situational dishonesty common in everyday life. Most people engage in this lying from time to time to avoid punishment, to protect someone's feelings, or simply for convenience. In contrast, pathological or habitual lying is a behavior characterized by a compulsive and persistent tendency to tell falsehoods, regardless of their significance or consequences. Individuals who engage in pathological lying routinely fabricate stories, exaggerate details, or present false information about various aspects of their lives. Unlike general lying, pathological lying appears to be driven by internal motivations unclear to the individual or those around them. It can strain relationships, erode trust, and have significant personal, social, and professional consequences. It is often considered a symptom of underlying psychological issues.[7,8]

Mom had a persistent habit of falsifying her achievements, financial status, employment history, and relationships, among other things. When it came to her financial struggles, she frequently shifted blame onto her marital partners or the financial responsibilities of "supporting" her adult children. She would exaggerate her job titles, such as claiming to work for "Target Corporation" and even carrying an elegant leather attaché case to work daily, despite her actual role being a fitting room attendant in a Target retail store. Her relationships and suspected extramarital affairs consistently deviated from reality in terms of their duration and trajectory. She'd say it was six months if she was with a guy for two months. As a child, she tried to convince me she was helping a married physician, her boss, study for boards … in a hotel room … by candlelight that she made me help set up. Her lies and gaslighting rarely worked on me. I could see through the nonsense but mostly had to stay silent. My motto now is "Believe nothing that you hear and half of what you see."

The sheer volume of Mom's falsehoods was staggering, making it impossible to recount them all. As a family, we mainly overlooked her tales unless they directly affected us. Engaging in daily confrontations would have been an endless and futile battle.

As my siblings and I grew older and into adulthood, Mom's tools of intimidation became less effective. We'd grown numb and mostly tuned her out. No longer our attention, Mom switched tactics—her new approach: emotional manipulation.

By its fundamental nature, emotional manipulation can be difficult to detect. Expressing genuine emotions like happiness, love, anger, or sadness is not a form of manipulation. However, it is problematic when someone uses emotions to get what they want from you. Emotional manipulation can occur in any interpersonal relationship with friends, coworkers, or family. The experience leaves you confused and causes you to question your sense of reality. It places the manipulator in the role of the victim, a classic narcissistic manipulation tactic.

Crying is an effective tool for emotional manipulation.[9] It can displace attention from the core issue and thrust everyone into savior mode. Tears trigger our need to pacify, appease, and rescue the person who appears to be physically in distress. Have you ever noticed how fast we search for facial tissue when another person cries? We tend to be uncomfortable with displays of grief and rush to make the crier feel better. We find it challenging to sit side by side when someone displays sorrow. Manipulative people understand it and use it to their advantage. They cry harder and louder to distract you from the truth. When weaponized, tears provide an endless way to avoid accountability and inhibit authentic communication.

Mom would start crying at the slightest touch. Questioning, contradicting, or ignoring her all led to the same outcome. Sobs sprung forth, instantly saturating her face. There were no degrees to it, no solitary tear, silent crying, or sniffling. It was always full out, heavy tears bouncing off of her cheeks. She'd get up and rush from the room or out the front door in feigned distress.

In her wake, her children immediately found themselves transformed into villains. It didn't matter if witnesses knew Mom was lying, attention-seeking, or insincere. We children had triggered tears and must be held accountable. It was easier to fall into that trap than to hold Mom responsible.

"Bridge, don't do that," my grandparents would chastise the young adult me. Maybe Mom had just told some fantastical tale of helping me pay for college or had lied about putting her phone bill in my name, not paying it, and ruining my credit. It didn't matter. My grandparents preferred maintaining the equilibrium, walking on eggshells to avoid setting Debra off.

I had empathy for my grandparents. They had to deal with Mom more regularly than I did. I was off at college and then graduate school, insulated from her daily antics. I knew that avoidance was a common and powerful defense mechanism. It was easier for my family to avoid the chaos than to confront Mom with the truth constantly. It may have seemed more straightforward and more effective to reprimand us, to take the path of least resistance. They weren't naïve or utterly blind to Mom's behavior. It's just how they coped.

When you know better, you do better. In graduate school, I was beginning to 'know' better. I could put a name to Mom's symptoms of NPD. I had the skills to assess the signs and accurately differentiate them from other disorders. I felt compelled to share it. I photocopied the pages of the *Diagnostic and Statistical Manual of Mental Disorders* and mailed it to my sister and grandparents with no explanation or attribution. Two days later, I got the first call.

"Whoa. This is deep. This is Debra exactly!" my grandparents agreed.

The revelation didn't always stick in their minds. They were used to handling Mom with delicacy and enabling her. It was still easier to avoid triggering her. It did give me and my siblings a more frequent reprieve from being blamed for Mom's crying episodes. Our grandparents started taking a more neutral stance, sometimes reminding us that Mom was unwell. Those pages that I'd sent brought the family a new reality. We couldn't change Mom; we could only change ourselves. It was progress. Maybe.

In time, Mom probably felt the family's desensitization to her outbursts. Her performances sometimes fell flat in the presence of a disinterested audience. Her spotlight had dimmed, and she needed a new way to re-center herself: cue, poor health.

References

1. Centers for Disease Control (CDC). (n.d.). *Fast facts: Preventing adverse childhood experiences.* https://www.cdc.gov/violenceprevention/aces/fastfact.html

2. American Psychiatric Association. (2022). Diagnostic and statistical manual of mental disorders. (5th ed., text rev.) https://doi.org/10.1176/appi.books.9780890425787

3. Mergui, J., Raveh, D., Gropp, C., Golmard, J.-L., & Jaworowski, S. (2015). Prevalence and characteristics of cluster B personality disorder in a consultation-liaison psychiatry practice. *International Journal of Psychiatry in Clinical Practice, 19*(1), 65–70. https://doi.org/10.3109/13651501.2014.981543

4. Kacel, E. L., Ennis, N., & Pereira, D. B. (2017). Narcissistic personality disorder in clinical health psychology practice: Case studies of comorbid psychological distress and life-limiting illness. *Behavioral Medicine (Washington, D.C.), 43*(3), 156–164. https://doi.org/10.1080/08964289.2017.1301875

5. Yeomans, F., & Caligor, E. (2016). Narcissistic personality disorder: The treatment challenge. *Psychiatrics News, 51*(9). https://doi.org/10.1176/appi.pn.2016.5a19

6. Franco, N. (2023, April). *Childhood roles developed in a narcissistic family.* https://nicolefrancocounseling.com/the-roles-we-play-in-a-narcissistic-family/

7. Curtis, D. A., & Hart, C. L. (2020). Pathological lying: Theoretical and empirical support for a diagnostic entity. *Psychiatric Research and Clinical Practice, 2*(2), 62–69. https://doi.org/10.1176/appi.prcp.20190046

8. Muzinic, L., Kozaric-Kovacic, D., & Marinic, I. (2016). Psychiatric aspects of normal and pathological lying. *International Journal of Law & Psychiatry, 46*, 88–93. https://doi.org/10.1016/j.ijlp.2016.02.036

9. van Roeyen, I., Riem, M. M. E., Toncic, M., & Vingerhoets, A. J. J. M. (2020). The damaging effects of perceived crocodile tears for a crier's image. *Frontiers in Psychology, 11*, 172. https://doi.org/10.3389/fpsyg.2020.00172

CHAPTER 13

I'm Starting to Feel Sick Tomorrow

Adverse Childhood Experience—Household Substance Abuse

Substance use refers to the consumption of specific substances, such as alcohol, tobacco, illicit drugs, inhalants, and other materials that can be ingested, inhaled, injected, or absorbed into the body, potentially leading to dependence and other harmful effects.[1]

IN MY FRESHMAN summer bridge program, my friends gave me the nickname *The Pharmacist*. At first, I was confused. Didn't everyone have a freezer bag full of medications tucked away in their dorm room, ready for any ailment? Headache? I had ibuprofen, acetaminophen, or a prescription-strength pain reliever. Stomach issues? Antacids, anti-nausea pills, or something stronger. Trouble sleeping? Take your pick. If someone needed something, I probably had it. Didn't we all?

To me, this was normal, mild even, compared to what I'd grown up with. But it was beginning to dawn on me that my family system was abnormal in more ways than I'd realized.

It wasn't until my new friend Sara, whose father was a physician, looked at me with a mix of curiosity and concern that I started to see it differently. She barely had anything in her dorm, maybe some aspirin or allergy pills, because, in her house, medications were kept only if they were prescribed for a specific reason.

"Where did you even get all this?" she asked one day, sifting through my bag, her voice laced with judgment.

The answer was simple: home.

Growing up, my mother's bottom dresser drawer was our household's unspoken apothecary. It overflowed with prescription bottles, some with her name, others with names I recognized as belonging to my grandparents, siblings, or aunts. There was a hierarchy to these medications, with narcotics holding a place of quiet reverence. She would talk about who had the *good stuff* after a surgery or hospital stay and how they *didn't need all of it.*

(dis)Honor Thy Mother: Daughterhood, Dysfunction and Deliverance, First Edition. Bridgette Peteet.
© 2026 John Wiley & Sons, Inc. Published 2026 by John Wiley & Sons, Inc.

I never questioned it. If my mother had a system, if she knew which pills worked for which symptoms, why would I think anything was wrong?

It wasn't until years later that I learned the term for this: prescription drug misuse. It exists on a spectrum, from occasional use outside medical guidelines to full-blown substance use disorder.[2] And while the dangers of illicit drugs were drilled into us at school and church, prescription drug misuse carried far less stigma. After all, these medications were given by doctors. They came in official bottles. They were meant to help.

But misuse is misuse, no matter how it's packaged. The risks—dependence, overdose, long-term health consequences—don't disappear just because a drug comes from a pharmacy instead of a street dealer. And yet, because prescription medications carry the authority of the medical system, people are often slow to recognize when casual use turns into something more dangerous.

Mom straddled that line. Her use was hidden in plain sight. She had smoked marijuana long before it was legalized. I could always smell it before I could see that she was high. But sometimes, there was something else. A shift in her, an intoxication without the familiar commingling scent of weed and perfume. That euphoric, drowsy look in her eye was difficult to explain before I knew what it was.

That look kept me reluctant to let her borrow my car one Friday night. I had to cheer for a basketball game, and she begged to use my car while I was there. Something felt off.

"No," I told her. "You seem high."

She scoffed. "I haven't smoked anything but cigarettes today."

I didn't believe her, but I also knew better than to push. She didn't have car insurance, but I didn't dare raise that issue either. Even though I was living with my grandparents, it was still difficult to resist my mother's authority.

I relented. She would drop me off at school across town and then take the car. We made it half a block.

Mom jumped the railroad tracks that sat atop a small hill, then slid straight through the stop sign at the intersection on the other side. A stop sign she had halted at for 38 years, down the street from her childhood home, except today. A blind spot in the poorly engineered roads of the South Side.

I saw the black sedan pause and continue forward with the right of way. I yelled, "STOP!"

But it was too late.

She clipped the back of the four-door, sending the other car spinning 90°. The driver was furious. I was furious. And then, quickly, I was afraid.

Mom pranced out of the car as if she were greeting an old friend. "Oh, it's fine. See?" she said, waving a dismissive hand as she wiped at the scratches with her sleeve.

I stood frozen, heart pounding. What if the other driver called the police? What if they realized what I now knew, Mom was high? Would they arrest her? Would they charge her for driving uninsured? Would they impound my car, leaving me stranded without transportation?

But with Mom's charm and manipulation, we were back in the car within minutes. This time, I insisted we switch seats. If she wanted to kill herself later on her own time, that was up to her. I had to protect myself.

***

In a performance of virtue seemingly meant to mask her disordered personality traits, Mom leaned into religion in her mid-40s. The day Mom got rebaptized she arrived in a rush, trailing the distinct scent of marijuana with constricted pupils likely from unprescribed prescription narcotics. She claimed to have experienced "racial profiling by the police" during her short commute to church. Racial profiling or suspected driving under influence (DUI)? I was skeptical.

Devon and I served as de facto deaconesses for our tiny home church that day, holding the white sheets out to collect Mom as she emerged from the baptismal pool. I searched for a transformation in her eyes. Instead, Mom cursed us for trying to "give [her] pneumonia" on account of our haste.

After her baptism, Mom blamed her sour fragrance on someone smoking near her—at her house. As medical marijuana laws began to pass in other states, she claimed to need it for her chronic health conditions. Which condition? I couldn't tell you.

At first, Mom's ailments were subtle. She complained of common medical conditions that were prevalent in our family. High blood pressure, bad knees, migraines, fibroids, and weight problems were par for the course. Pretty much everyone in the family over the age of 30 had at least two of these illnesses. The "new knees" were a running joke and a glim reality in our family of former athletes. Mom was a little different. She claimed them all, which at first wasn't particularly unusual. Then, it became too technical, too fast, and too much.

Early in 2007, Uncle Brian, Mom's brother, was diagnosed with sleep apnea. He saw a specialist and had gone through an intense overnight sleep study. The technicians likely monitored his brain waves, eye movements, heart rate, blood oxygen levels, body positioning, and breathing patterns. After his diagnosis, he was given a continuous positive airway pressure (CPAP) machine to help maintain his breathing overnight. Immediately after sharing his news, Mom announced that she, too, had sleep apnea. No specialist. No study. No intervention. She just declared it.

That spring, my nephew fell off the monkey bars at the park. His mom, Devon, rushed him to urgent care. He had sprained his ankle and came home in an ankle wrap. Later that same day, Mom said she had a "bad sprain" too. Devon reported that Mom wrapped her ankle up, laid down, and propped her foot up on a pillow. There were no details of when or how she fell and no witnesses.

That summer, I was far into my pregnancy with my first child, and I'd had sciatic nerve pain since the second trimester. One morning, I bent over to change the bedroom trash and threw my back out completely. I was frozen at a 90° angle, belly to lap, for three days. By some "twintuition," 1.5 hours away, Mom shared that she was also suffering from sciatica. The pattern was becoming clear.

Around the same time, Uncle Brian shared that his then-wife was diagnosed with Addison's disease, a rare illness characterized by low hormones and flares that can cause life-threateningly low blood pressure. Mom wrote me a long letter informing me that she had Addison's. No specialist had taken blood tests of her sodium, potassium, or cortisol levels, nor had she received any treatment. She just stated it as fact and asked me not to tell her parents, seemingly to provide a shroud of validating secrecy. Granny and I were close, though, and we talked about almost everything. We routinely corroborated any stories Mom told to uncover the near truth. Mom had already told Granny this allegedly "devastating" health news; in the same vein, she'd told Granny not to tell us.

Alarm bells were ringing everywhere—four ailments copied from other family members in quick succession. Yet again, I questioned my sense of reality. Mom routinely accused me of being "too hard on her." Was it me?

I was a licensed clinical psychologist by then, but Mom's manipulations were so longstanding and powerful that I still didn't fully trust my perceptions of her. The family was on the fence, too. It is difficult to speak out against someone feigning illnesses without appearing unempathetic and cold. We were conservative in our responses to her and mildly supportive as each new ailment emerged. Mom had our emotions in a chokehold. Facts, on the other hand, couldn't be disputed as easily. It had worked once to ground us the printouts of those pages of the *DSM*. So, I created a log.

I swiped a long sheet of paper used for grocery lists from the front of the refrigerator and started keeping a record. Calls, emails, letters, texts, and hearsay reports of Mom's professed illnesses made the dated list that I kept casually in my nightstand drawer:

"… kidney tissue infection,"
"… took a bad fall,"
"… 80% deaf in my right ear,"
"… going through a second menopause, which explains all the crying,"
"… stress threw my blood pressure up into stroke zones,"

"… had to ask Devon to wash my hair because I am experiencing numbness on my left side,"

"… Doctors are worried about the big C."

"… I scored an 18 on a test for fibromyalgia where only 11 points are needed for a diagnosis,"

I delivered my first child in August of that year and had what the nurses jokingly called a "vaginal C-section" (not funny at the time). As the doctor was sewing me up, for what felt like days, my mother lamented that she had torn even worse than me during her own childbirths yet, in reality, she had delivered all of us by cesarean.

Soon after, Granny had a rare simultaneous double knee replacement surgery. The family huddled around the heavily sedated 72-year-old patient. There was nowhere to sit because Mom had created a makeshift bed out of two chairs. She'd stolen Granny's post-surgical compression socks and moaned, "both of my knees are blown out."

This was the first year alone. In that time, Mom had never been to the emergency room, been hospitalized, or had any known procedures. Though she had doctor-shopped until someone told her what she wanted to hear, she called the other doctors who questioned her "quacks." She eventually found one doctor who allegedly practiced holistic medicine. She wrote me another letter saying, "It's a relief to finally get confirmed that I'm indeed not out of my head or making up pains" and went on to summarize the doctor's one-visit findings:

"… blood clot in my brain that could kill me at any second,"

"… headed to see a neurosurgeon today,"

"… rheumatoid arthritis,"

"… malaria,"

"… the bubonic plague."

This is no exaggeration. Mom claimed to have contracted the black death. Between 2007 and 2013, the front and back sides of the page had grown to 30 serious illnesses. That's an average of four major health problems annually. It included deadly, rare diseases requiring intensive medical intervention tracking and hospitalizations Mom had never had. She was sick, but not with any of the various illnesses she'd believed.

Psychologically, Mom's symptoms were consistent with a factitious disorder. A factitious disorder is a serious mental illness where someone fakes, exaggerates, or induces medical problems and diseases for themselves or others with no apparent external reward (e.g., to get out of work).[3] You may have heard of or seen movies about Munchausen syndrome by proxy, which is when a parent or caretaker exaggerates, makes up, or induces fake symptoms in their children.[4] When it is self-inflicted, it is called Munchausen syndrome or factitious disorder.

The underlying drive for either tends to be acquiring sympathy, affection, and attention. These individuals tend to doctor-shop to support their claims and to obtain prescription drugs or medical treatment. They may work to appear sick by losing weight or shaving their hair. The disorder is more prevalent among healthcare professionals.[5]

People with certain personality disorders, like the narcissistic personality disorder (NPD) (previously discussed), are more susceptible to factitious disorders. Unlike psychosis, where individuals are intermittently or permanently detached from reality, there is a degree of consciousness and control with these types of disorders. People with these syndromes understand human behavior at a primal level and have learned to manipulate emotions with ease. Some of their actions are impulsive and difficult to control, and some are calculated planned behavior. Much like personality disorders, factitious disorders are nearly impossible to treat.

I was beginning to accept that Mom couldn't change. Her issues were deep rooted, untreatable, and permanent. I finally got what it was; it was hard to grasp why. I wanted to understand how she came to have these complex pathologies.

Psychologists theorize and study the cause of psychological disorders. The nature–nurture debate is ongoing, genetics versus early environmental influences. It is usually a combination of both factors.

Many psychiatric disorders tend to run in families, suggesting a biological basis. The odds of having a specific disorder are higher if other relatives have the illness. However, inheritance does not always manifest linearly, meaning psychological disorders don't automatically pass from parent to child. It can occur multiple times in one generation or even skip generations.

This may be the case in my family. From their accounts, Granny and Pawpaw's mothers exhibited signs of mental disorders like my mother. My great-grandmothers are described as being angry, impulsive, and emotionally unstable. Both relinquished their maternal responsibilities to others, which was uncommon in the 1930s and 1940s. Of course, neither was ever formally diagnosed. The first edition of the *DSM* wasn't even published until 1952,[6] but their behavior hints at a family history of mental illness.

Considering nurture, environmental factors leading to mental illness are attributable to adverse childhood experiences (ACEs), including trauma, emotional abuse, or exposure to drugs and alcohol. These issues were not present in my grandparents' highly religious household. Though imperfect, they strived to instill values of discipline, compassion, honesty, and personal responsibility. However, these values didn't seem to stick for some of their offspring, and the extremes of emotional volatility, self-centeredness, dishonesty, and entitlement prevailed. In a war against genetics, they lost many battles.

Specific to personality disorders, some experts suggest that parents offering too much or too little adoration and praise that is disproportionate to the child's experience or accomplishments may contribute to developing personality disorders. This may be most fitting. My grandparents believed themselves infertile after being unable to conceive during the first four years of their marriage. Infertility was heavily stigmatized in those days. When Mom finally arrived, she was favored within the nuclear and extended family, Granny is said to have treated her like a human doll, clothing her in the prettiest dresses, taking countless pictures, and doting on her. Mom was considered a "Daddy's girl" and her role as the "princess" was more firmly solidified when the successive biological children were male. Like most men of that era, Pawpaw was known to be a lot harder on the boys in the family. My uncles say Mom "got away with murder" as they all endeavored to be the picture-perfect family.

Mom calls her childhood experiences "trauma." Though she favored this phrase, her descriptions do not meet the mark. In one 17-page letter, Mom wrote me about her "personal hell" growing up. She penned that she was an "awesome child and was better than good." She invited me to imagine "NEVER getting any credit when you desperately needed someone to believe you and in you." Ultimately, Mom believes she didn't get as much attention and admiration as she deserved, but that isn't trauma or parental child abuse. Her need for constant validation did sound familiar though (see Chapter 12).

Looking to a more objective measure than self-report, we return to the ACEs assessment. Of the ten original categories of abuse, Mom may or may not have had one. At about age 60, she began frequently reporting that she'd been sexually abused as a child by an older relative. Mom had a habit of fabricating stories, so it wasn't easy to ascertain whether it was truthful. It followed her usual pattern of deflection and melodramatic escalation.

Mom's story of abuse first emerged when Devon disclosed that Mom's 3rd husband, Ricky, had abused her. Centering the narrative on her victimization seemed a way for Mom to absolve her guilt for exposing her child to a known predator. It carelessly minimized the severity of Devon's abuse by framing it as ordinary or insignificant. This response is not exceptionally uncommon. Some of my patients have reported that their mothers didn't believe their stories of sexual abuse, and in many cases, including Devon's, the woman stays with the offender. This may be due to the mother's experience of emotional abuse, financial dependence on the offender, or desire for companionship.

Mom was offended that we didn't immediately condemn and exile her accused abuser when she began sharing her story with more frequency and flair. She felt that he should no longer be included in family events and that we were "retraumatizing" her by inviting him. She claimed she'd always been uncomfortable around him, but that wasn't evident.

I recalled our family visiting this distant relative when I was in my 20s. Six of us, Mom, boyfriend, and children, had crashed in the living room of our relative's small two-bedroom apartment. In the morning, we were taking turns getting dressed in the single bathroom. Meanwhile, Mom started ironing her clothes in the common area. The problem was that she only wore a black lacey bra and matching slip. I was shocked at the social faux pas.

"Mom, put a shirt on!" I rebuked with a parental tone that I'd perfected in dealing with her by then.

"Whatever, Bridgette. Don't be so uptight!" Mom snaked her neck, waved me off, and continued her chore.

Reflecting on that experience in the context of Mom's allegations toward that same relative, I couldn't reconcile the divergent images. *Would I or anyone else stand in someone's home in lingerie let alone if they had abused me?* To me, it would be inappropriate to do as a guest in anyone's home. I couldn't see anyone doing this in front of someone who had been sexually abusive.

Mom began to share her story anytime she had an audience. She told coworkers she barely knew as she hopped from job to job. She shared it with acquaintances and family friends, the gossip all quickly twisting back through the small-town grapevine. She ultimately stood up before the church congregation and testified. Jaws dropped when she added that her parents "knew and did nothing about [her abuse]." My grandparents were hurt, humiliated, and utterly defenseless against Mom's accusations. All they had to rely on was their reputation versus hers.

Behaviorally, the evidence that this was a significant trauma didn't align. There were no other reports of victimization in the family. There were no efforts to reduce or impede contact with this relative. However, statistically, something of this nature could have happened to Mom. More than half (51%) of women have been touched sexually without their permission in their lifetime.[7–9] One in four women and one in six men have experienced childhood sexual abuse. It is a huge problem and a common secret held within families.

We'll never know what really happened. I only feel comfortable pointing out the pattern of escalation that I've witnessed; however, I am fully confident that whatever the case, it does not match the severity and multiplicity of my mother's illnesses. Most abused people do not go on to be abusive. Her ever-winding pursuit of victimization is a sign rather than the source of her pathology.

***

I was visiting my Uncle Brian at his home in Florida in the fall of 2018. My uncle and I have always been close. He was always the humorous Uncle, the youngest of Granny and Pawpaw's biological children. By his own account, he'd been somewhat reckless in his youth but had turned his life around. He joined the military and raised a family. In his mid-30s, he went to college and graduated the year before me. He was the first one brave enough to challenge the family status quo. To call out the crazy. Literally. He was the one who'd made that anonymous report to child protective services (CPS) when we were children. He helped save us.

Uncle Brian passed me his cell phone, displaying a lengthy message thread from Mom. As I continued to scroll and scroll, her words followed the usual convoluted path, drifting from one topic to another. The beginning scenario didn't involve her, but she was dead center by the end, ultimately reaching the subject of her alleged abuse.

"Mom and Dad didn't protect me then or now! You all expect me to be around my abusers with no questions. I've always been uncomfortable."

"Abusers," plural, caught my attention. She'd added an -s-. Her accusations had expanded with one letter. Confused, I kept scrolling.

"Bridgette and Devon are always attacking me. I have witnesses. Malik and my friends have had to shield me and take me away from their torment countless times."

My grip tightened on the outer edges of the cell phone case. Bridgette and Devon were the dynamic duo. We'd somehow become Mom's "abusers" instead of vice versa. We were like the Kevin Bacons in Mom's narratives; only instead of six degrees of separation, there was one and all roads led to us. All bad things were our fault.

Emotionally, the lies got under my skin. Cognitively and clinically, I understood it. Due to Mom's mental illness, her world was black and white. Those closest to her were all good or bad depending on how well they served her, a psychological term called *splitting*. Their position was set based on the potency of the narcissistic fix they provided her. She gravitated toward those who enabled her. She shunned and disparaged those who called her out or refused to engage.

By that point, Devon and I hadn't had an in-depth interaction with Mom in five years. We had been pressured to reconcile with her time after time. Familial and religious guilt to "honor" our mother pushed us back into her toxic embrace for 20 years since the first time I'd run at age 15. This was the longest we'd held our ground.

With our distance, new flashes of insight began to emerge in the family. Uncle Brian could now see that it didn't make sense that Devon and I remained central figures in Mom's stories. He shut her down when she began suggesting that Granny, his mother, had a mental illness. He was an eyewitness to the illogical nature of her accusations. He began to accept that her behavior was not a temporary state. He apologized for ever pressuring us to reengage with her. It was as if he'd fully weighed the facts and offered an informal diagnosis.

"She's really lost it," he offered me helplessly.

"Yeah, I know," I cosigned.

A Narcissist's Prayer

That didn't happen.

And if it did, it wasn't that bad.

And if it was, that's not a big deal.

And if it is, that's not my fault.

And if it was, I didn't mean it.

And if I did, you deserved it.

—Dayna Craig

References

1. Centers for Disease Control and Prevention (CDC). (n.d.). *Fast facts: Preventing adverse childhood experiences.* https://www.cdc.gov/violenceprevention/aces/fastfact.html

2. Rockhill, K. M., Olson, R., Dart, R. C., Iwanicki, J. L., & Black, J. C. (2023). Differing behaviors around adult non-medical use of prescription stimulants and opioids: Latent class analysis. *Journal of Medical Internet Research, 25*, e46742. https://doi.org/10.2196/46742

3. American Psychiatric Association (APA). (2022). Diagnostic and statistical manual of mental disorders (5th ed., text rev.). https://doi.org/10.1176/appi.books.9780890425787

4. Day, L. B., Faust, J., Black, R. A., Day, D. O., & Alexander, A. (2017). Personality profiles of factitious disorder imposed by mothers: A comparative analysis. *Journal of Child Custody, 14*(2/3), 191–208. https://doi.org/10.1080/15379418.2017.1331780

5. Yates, G. P., & Feldman, M. D. (2016). Factitious disorder: A systematic review of 455 cases in the professional literature. *General Hospital Psychiatry, 41*, 20–28. https://doi.org/10.1016/j.genhosppsych.2016.05.002

6. American Psychiatric Association (APA) (1952). *Diagnostic and statistical manual of mental disorders*. Washington DC: American Psychiatric Association.

7. Finkelhor, D., Shattuck, A., Turner, H. A., & Hamby, S. L. (2014). The lifetime prevalence of child sexual abuse and sexual assault assessed in late adolescence. *Journal of Adolescent Health*, *55*(3), 329–333. https://doi.org/10.1016/j.jadohealth.2013.12.026

8. Finkelhor, D., Turner, H., & Colburn, D. (2024). The prevalence of child sexual abuse with online sexual abuse added. *Child Abuse & Neglect*, *149*, 106634. https://doi.org/10.1016/j.chiabu.2024.106634

9. Gewirtz-Meydan, A., & Finkelhor, D. (2020). Sexual abuse and assault in a large national sample of children and adolescents. *Child Maltreatment*, *25*(2), 203–214. https://doi.org/10.1177/1077559519873975

CHAPTER 14

Cardiac Arrest

> Adverse Childhood Experience—Emotional Neglect
>
> *Child emotional neglect as the failure to meet a child's emotional needs, which include having feelings validated and responded to appropriately.*[1]

I WAS STARTLED out of my light slumber. Was it the thick heat of that August morning or the sharp ache in my lower abdomen that had startled me awake that day? Heat or pain, it didn't matter. It had my attention.

I'd had contractions for six hours the week before, only to eventually be told that it was Braxton Hicks or false labor.

"What's the difference, and how will I know it's real?" I asked the nurse.

She quipped, "You'll have a baby at the end of one."

Not amusing.

It was my first baby. My July 31 due date had long passed—every day after felt like an extra week. Damien's family kept saying it would be "sweet" if I had our daughter on his birthday, August 18. That sounded like torture. It was already August 10. There was no room left in the inn. This baby needed to come out.

I could no longer turn over in bed alone or get up from low chairs without Damien heaving my 200+ lb into a new position. With record heat days above 90° that summer, I'd retained so much water that even flip-flops were too tight.

I'd researched natural remedies and took everything to no avail. Spicy food gave me heartburn. Castor oil and orange juice, well, made things slick. I disliked tea, but raspberry leaf became my new drink of choice. Nothing. She was stuck like a pit in a peach.

(dis)Honor Thy Mother: Daughterhood, Dysfunction and Deliverance, First Edition. Bridgette Peteet.
© 2026 John Wiley & Sons, Inc. Published 2026 by John Wiley & Sons, Inc.

The next electric jolt catapulted me upright in the bed; no assistance was needed. The clock read that it was 4:32 a.m. If this were false labor again, I wouldn't make it.

Damien would have to go to work in a few hours and needed rest. There was no need to wake him if it was another false alarm. I could hold off for two hours. I gave myself a mental gold star at every 11-minutes increment that I endured. I held my breath for the 30 seconds or so of discomfort, curling into a fetal position on my side of the bed and trying not to horse-kick Damien in the back.

By 6:15 a.m., my effort felt sufficient. I reached over and backhanded Damien's chest far more aggressively than intended. He jumped up, out of bed, and landed, positioned with his arms and legs wide as if he were about to catch a football.

"I think I'm in labor," I shrieked.

He stood up straighter and side-eyed me.

"Are you sure?"

"No!" I breathed heavily.

"How far apart are your contractions?"

"I think 8 minutes, but I lost track."

That was his job now.

"Should we call the doctor?" Damien asked after watching my face contort at regular intervals.

"We have to wait until 9:00, or there's an after-hours fee."

It felt like the clock was moving backward, farther away from the hour than closer. At 8:59 a.m., I inhaled, hit autodial on my cell phone, and prayed that someone was in the office on time.

As soon as the line answered, I blurted out my information, name, date of birth, doctor's name, length, and space of contractions. The nurse on the other end was too calm for my taste. It was as if she'd gotten this call hundreds of times before from first-time mothers, but this was my first rodeo. The pain was hitting differently. This was the real thing: an emergency! Only it wasn't. Women have given birth since Eve. I wasn't unique. I could tell. The nurse coolly directed me to go to the emergency room at the hospital where I was supposed to deliver.

Sixteen hours from start to finish, they heaved her, covered in what resembled raw chicken skin, atop my chest. My heart skipped a beat. Taryn was perfect. I'd gotten no credit for my long labor; she looked like her daddy with powdery skin and curly jet-black hair. It'd be almost three years before redemption came with Jordyn, our second girl who looked just like me with brown skin and dark brown hair. She'd be my mini me and shadow, born on my birthday, no less.

I can still recall those first feelings of motherhood with Taryn, though. My heart swelled to an unfamiliar capacity, instantly full as I looked into her dark eyes. That little 8th of her right iris that wanted to be hazel. I loved her.

Emotion hit me like a tsunami, and I began to sob, my body shaking. Maybe it was the anesthesia wearing off. I don't know, but something about my emotions felt unhinged, out of control. It was like I was being washed over some mental cliff, the brink of something unknown and difficult, if not impossible, to return from. Mentally, I visualized clawing my way back up, newborn in tow, and grounding myself back in the present.

I steadied, ready for the challenging road of motherhood ahead. One for which there was no blueprint, but one that I'd considered since middle school, vowing that my future children would have a different life than I'd had.

I touched Taryn's palm, and she gripped my pointer finger tightly.

I bet she rocked that newborn Apgar test, good color, pulse, response to stimulation, muscle tone, and respiration. Advanced already.

I took in her size as she seemed to sprawl completely across my chest. *How had she fit inside of me?* She was huge. I see why it'd been so hard to get her out.

Eight pounds and change. The metal forceps used to retrieve her had ripped me to shreds. The doctor was still sewing.

I stroked her tiny head, misshapen from birth, and her hat lifted. Just above her right eyebrow was a tiny, crimson cut.

Who hurt her? How? Why didn't they say anything? Was it the forceps?

I felt like getting off the table and fighting the guilty one. If only my legs weren't sedated and the doctor wasn't busy stitching my two halves back together. I asked most of these questions aloud. The nurse assured me the medical devices were dull, but no one could account for my baby's wound. The nurse brought over some ointment and a long cotton swab to appease me.

"I'll do it," I seethed, taking the supplies from her outstretched hands.

Motherhood sent me to a new level of assertiveness, more confident and fearless in my beliefs. New, unfamiliar primal maternal instincts set in. It was automatic, though I acknowledge that it's not like that for everyone. I would die to protect my two daughters.

Motherhood was nothing like *she'd* prophesized. *You'll understand me better when you have kids*, Mom had always promised. It felt like more of a threat than hope.

I kept waiting; years passed. Understanding never came. Motherhood made me understand my mom even less.

Don't get me wrong; I did gain a new appreciation of the labor and exhaustion that goes into parenting. The everyday stressors of childrearing are not easy. The lack of adequate support inside the home and limited financial resources would have made it even more difficult for my mother. It wasn't any of that.

I had a fierce urge to protect my daughters from harm, sacrifice for their benefit, and provide unconditional love. My girls would be supervised. We would put their needs ahead of our own. We would love them no matter what they did. We would provide a constant and safe bubble, not just from the outside world, but from *anyone* that might cause them harm intentionally or not. I was unapologetic in protecting and loving my daughters.

***

As homecoming night approached, I could feel the buzz of excitement in the air. It would be my daughter Taryn's first dance, the most anticipated evening of her high school life thus far. She'd fallen in love with her new high school, having amnesia over the meltdown at the prospect of transferring after her first year at her parents' suggestion.

She'd been withering on the vine and was now thriving in the new environment, not just in her usual academic endeavors. Taryn bonded with her varsity basketball teammates over the summer tournament season. Her well-trained teachers were more engaging and supportive, and Taryn was stepping into student leadership roles where she'd been invisible the year before. A month and a half into the school year, Taryn surprised me with her new-found excitement for school activities. It was homecoming.

Our trio of mother–daughter dyads had traipsed around nearby cities on the hunt for the perfect gown for each of our girls. Taryn and I were momentarily swept up in the enthusiasm of $300 dresses but eventually calmed and settled on an off-the-rack royal blue gown with a purple sequin overlay that fit her like a glove. I'd scoured the internet for the perfect shoe, finding one with a coordinating iridescent shade of purple and a comfortable low-block heel.

As her reluctant hairdresser, I tried and failed several times to create a style to appease my simplistic-minded teenager. Ultimately, I twisted the top half of her long locs into two connecting fishtail braids at the back of her head, forming a crown. I'd scrolled through 41 Pinterest pages for eyeshadow tutorials and attempted to recreate the artistic strokes meant for professionals. Art had always been my worst subject. Taryn pushed me to modify and tone down the looks. She was way too overconfident in my abilities.

My rainbow-colored starburst earrings coordinated perfectly with the teardrop necklace I'd found for her on Amazon. My purple, shimmery evening bag finished the look. I stepped back, admiring the finished product as she examined herself in the mirror. My heart swelled two sizes with affection for my daughter as I looked at her reflection. She was ready to fly.

"You look beautiful!" I said to my daughter.

***

"You look beautiful," I said, trying to find sincerity.

It was July 4th, 2003, our wedding day. My friend Ebony, also a bridesmaid, was applying a thin coat of makeup to my face. We were shrouded in a small nursing room just outside the church sanctuary, where three other bridesmaids and our wedding planner were adding the final touches to our simple yet elegant affair.

Against my wishes, my mother had somehow managed to barge into the room. I hadn't wanted her there. From the beginning, she had done everything she could to undermine my wedding plans. She'd hastily become engaged to her fourth husband just a week after we'd announced our engagement. On a nonexistent budget, her gilded dreams for her wedding had caused a tantrum because she "wanted ooohs and ahhs over [her] stuff too." She said she would "let me have purple" since it was my "first wedding."

Amid my planning, she'd wedded. Then, at the last minute, she insisted we hire her new husband as our bridal photographer despite our having already paid a nonrefundable deposit to a professional. She called us "selfish" when we refused, a classic psychological projection. She'd even demanded that her husband of just six months walk her down the aisle and be in photos because my stepmother, Tamara, who had been part of my life for 13 years, was granted the honor.

By the time our nuptials arrived, I needed some distance from her. So, when she pushed her way into the room, I held my breath, bracing for what might come next.

Mom's first words weren't a simple "hi," "hello," or even "congratulations." Instead, she remarked, "You didn't tell me I look beautiful!"

Mom couldn't walk past a mirror without looking at herself. It was as if it was a portal to a world where she could transform herself into the idealized image she held in her mind, a world where her beauty, real or imagined, was celebrated and revered. She'd once swerved into the right lane on the highway, earning a startling honk from an irate semi-truck driver high above.

"Yes sir, I know I'm fine," Mom retorted.

In the passenger seat, I whipped my head back and forth in confusion. There was no way he could've seen her face. She'd encroached on his lane, but her perception was that her unparalleled beauty was the cause of the commotion.

The church nursery room fell into an uneasy hush, eyes darting in disbelief, bridesmaids ready to pounce if called. Faced with a choice between escalation and de-escalation, I opted for peace and consented to her request. I told her that she looked beautiful. Unfortunately, it did little to halt the drama.

Later that evening, during an activity at the reception, Mom commandeered the microphone to offer us marital advice as a "newlywed" herself. The following day, we had planned a potluck after church, and Mom was responsible for preparing the main dish, a large lasagna, and her sole contribution to the weekend's festivities. To our bewilderment, she abruptly left without informing us, leaving our guests hungry and angry … at us.

Granny had called Mom's overall behavior toward me "jealousy," but I didn't comprehend envy from a mother toward her daughter. They say parents are the only people who want you to do better than them. It's the natural order of things. I couldn't grasp anything to the contrary.

I was determined that my daughters would have a different kind of mother: supportive, nurturing, noncompetitive. I would work to be a healthy but not all-sacrificing type. In their elementary school years, I alternated my service as the "Room Mom" for each child yearly. I stretch my artistic abilities to make them special homemade birthday cakes ranging from Barbie dolls to beach themes. I attend every one of their games, performances, and award ceremonies that my schedule and energy allow. I sit with them almost every night in our bedroom and listen to the recap of their day.

It is also essential for me to make time for self-care. I love the spa and try to go biannually. To maintain our physical health, Damien and I go to the gym in alternating shifts, him early in the morning and me in the evening. I maintain social connections with friends and even joined an alumnae sorority chapter to complement my ongoing community service. I am determined to break the cycle of ACEs and give my daughters a childhood filled with love, stability, and security.

At times, I felt uncomfortable violating norms in my family of origin. As a licensed clinical psychologist, my family didn't recognize that I had additional insights that informed my decisions. I knew the importance of emotional connection, positive, healthy touch, nurturing, and secure attachments.[2] Behaviorally, I was aware of the benefits of schedules, predictability, and stability. I'd counseled and personally lived through the damaging effects of neglect, physical abuse, and emotional torment. I had the desire and knowledge to do something different.

Within the first months of motherhood, these perspectives collided. It was Thanksgiving, and we visited my in-laws' extended family in Detroit. Everyone who hadn't met her was eager and excited to see the new baby. I sat her infant car seat on the kitchen floor and unzipped the fluffy cover to reveal her sleeping face. The family gathered around. I understood the draw as Taryn had one of those angelic faces that made strangers want to touch her. Without asking, one relative crouched down to unbuckle her.

I intervened. "Oh no, it's her nap time. You can hold her when she wakes up."

Maybe the fatigue of sleep training put unintentionally and unconsciously sharp edges on my words. Perhaps the strain of traveling out of state by car for four hours with a newborn hadn't left me at my best. In my mind, I was smiling and gentle in my redirection. But, speechless, the cousin-by-marriage recoiled like she'd been burned. She started crying and left the room. I figured something else was happening with her that day, but later, I heard her telling the family that I "hated" her. I was shocked that I was the cause of her tears when it was really about my baby's well-being. It was about our family maintaining our sanity despite extreme sleep deprivation. Sleep is excellent medicine. It benefits your physical and mental health. It wasn't about her at all. I could've conveyed that part out loud, but that wasn't my strength. I process a lot internally and sometimes forget to clue other people in. This sometimes causes unintended conflict.

About three years later, we were visiting family. Some of the extended cousins were invited for a sleepover. At least six adults, including my husband, begged and pleaded for me to let Taryn stay over. I was resolved. The answer was an unequivocal no. The reasons seemed evident to me. The family did not take it well, which was an extremely awkward exchange.

Later, in private, I could explain to my husband that I'd been pulled into a family consultation with the sleepover hosts about their oldest child earlier that day. They'd just been called into a parent–teacher meeting because their 1st-grader was putting dolls into sexually suggestive positions. As I advised the family, that is atypical for a child of that age and could be a sign that the child had been abused. It seemed absurd that they would then turn around and ask me to let my toddler spend the night. My decision wasn't out of spite but out of an abundance of caution. I was keeping my daughter safe.

Shielding my children vicariously trained me to guard myself and share my true thoughts and opinions. My people-pleasing tendency lessened. I had a voice, and I started to use it. Had I swung too far in the opposite direction? Maybe, but here's how it might go.

- *One of my dad's sisters might feel inclined to comment on her niece's weight gain while neglecting her own at a holiday gathering. I might offer facts about the detrimental effects of weight shaming on people's self-esteem.*
- *A grandpa might critique me for being nontraditional and failing as a wife because I don't iron Damien's work shirts. I might respectfully remind him that both members of our household work full-time and that egalitarian relationships are the new norm.*

- *Please, dear relative, don't refer to my children's hair as "good." All hair is good, and this idea reinforces divisive rhetoric within the Black community.*
- *No cousin, it's probably not a good idea to marry a girlfriend struggling with addiction for apparent reasons.*
- *Ma'am, you can't have a career in massage therapy if you have debilitating arthritis.*
- *Yeah, it's probably going to keep escalating if you let an abusive person move back in.*
- *Girl, when has getting pregnant to lock a man down ever been an effective strategy?*
- *Dude, using someone's credit card without permission is a crime.*

The generational curse that forced us into silent consent no longer bound me. I remained respectful, never yelling, never combative, but resisting with facts and likely endings. I didn't go around casting judgment anymore or offering unsolicited advice, but if asked, I'd try to be honest and helpful. However, I am careful to remember that my opinions sometimes carry more weight than I intend. For example, sometimes I can't casually say, "That's crazy," without someone taking it literally. People hear the psychologist speaking when sometimes it's just Bridgette. Bridgette is more flip and operates top of mind. Dr. Peteet is more empathetic and conscientious about her words. It's mostly that much of what I say doesn't seem that profound to me. It feels like simple cause and effect.

Choosing wisely seems natural to me. I forget that it's not for everyone. They say "a smart person learns from their own mistakes, and a wise person learns from the mistakes of others." My insights likely come from a combination of a childhood that required me to constantly observe the world and years of professional training and practice. That doesn't mean choosing perfectly, though. Insight and sound decision-making don't free you from all mistakes or shield you from the uncontrollable things in life (e.g., other people, the economy, natural disasters). It just helps you to move down a less dramatic and traumatic path on a more consistent basis. I believe that our choices account for much of the variability in the quality of our lives. It is invaluable to think through our options and the likely outcomes to make informed decisions. I've learned that the choices that offer instant gratification or are not grounded in reality will not work out in the long run. You cannot simply think for now but must also consider the future.

You also teach people how to treat (or mistreat) you by what you permit in your life. Setting limits for what you will and will not tolerate is psychologically healthy. Expressing your emotions and expecting them to be honored is valid. It is not always an easy transition to set new boundaries. People don't like it when you switch up the game. They may get upset, name-call, avoid, and generally resist the new rules of engagement. That's normal, but resisting the temptation to back down is important. The consistency of your actions re-trains people on how to engage with you in healthy ways. It may take them some time to adapt; many will, while others will not.

With my mother, I started setting new boundaries with incrementally firmer consequences. Initial violations were met with reminders. I might say, "Please don't talk about me." If it continued, I'd say "I don't want to get into it with you. Can we please talk about something else?" If my mother were going to be in attendance, I'd ensure that my emotional buffers were present. These included Damien, Devon, and sometimes Granny. At a minimum, they were witnesses. If necessary, they'd deflect her attacks and protect me. My children, husband, and I would leave in the worst situations. I recognize that we are privileged in that. We didn't rely on my mother or family for economic or childcare support. They had no leverage to draw us back in against our will. As things continued, we limited our engagement. Mom liked to send texts so long that you had to scroll up on your screen three times to get through it, letters the length of short stories, and one-sided calls lasting almost an hour. I'd send brief responses to her texts. I'd have Damien read her letters and report anything I needed to hear. I screened her calls for times when I was in the mental capacity to handle it. That's as far as I intended for it to go, but it wasn't enough. I was taking wise advice from friends and learning to protect my peace at all costs. I would eventually pay the full price.

***

*Ding.

I picked up my cell phone off of the couch next to me. The text message preview showed that it was a message from Mom. Against my will, my eyes rolled toward the ceiling.

What's she about to say?

I unlocked my phone and clicked to read the message.

"Pawpaw doesn't have a pulse."

My heart froze.

Pawpaw's dead!

How?

What happened?

No!

I couldn't believe it. Pawpaw had lived a respectable 80 years since his birth in 1933. For more than six decades, he was Granny's partner—her anchor and, at times, her storm. She had always said she wanted to "go first," convinced her heart couldn't endure the loss of the man she had loved for most of her life. Even after all those years, she said her heart still skipped a beat whenever she saw him.

Their story spanned lifetimes, starting when Granny was just a teenager. She bore him three children, raised three others and then opened their home to us, their grandchildren. Through it all, she stood beside him, even when whispers of his disloyalty reached her ears or when his tall tales and old-school chauvinism tested her patience. She endured.

Pawpaw wasn't perfect—no one is—but there was greatness in him all the same. His stoicism, his resilience, and the way he could fill a room with his presence left an undeniable mark on all of us. He was a man of his time, shaped by the world he was born into, yet loved deeply by the family he helped build. His flaws were a part of him, but they didn't overshadow the foundation of love and strength that defined his life and his legacy.

Granny and I were close, more like mother and daughter, and similar to one another in our struggles to overcome imperfect childhoods. Granny fueled my love for reading even though she had a 10th-grade education. I'd help her with words she didn't understand, and she helped me understand life. She taught me to cook, and I taught her multiplication. She took me to church and helped me realize that there was something out there bigger than me and that I was built for a particular purpose. I was her favorite, maybe to compensate for the fact that I was my mother's least favorite. She'd say she didn't mean to favor me; it was just that she didn't have to worry about me as much as the others. She was my safe person, and I was hers. With the news of Pawpaw, I had to get to her. She'd need me.

I hit the phone icon to call Mom back, and three rings. No answer. I tried again, but nothing. I hit redial again, and my impatience grew with each incessant ring. The last time, I let it ring four times. She finally picked up.

Thank goodness.

"Hi, this is Debra. I'm not available...."

Voicemail? Really?! I pressed the red icon to end the call.

Why isn't she answering? Ughhhhh!!!!

I tried Granny and Pawpaw's cell phone next. It was Sabbath, and they would've been leaving after church activities that Saturday afternoon. Their phone would have likely been powered off and buried in the depths of Granny's massive handbag, "pocketbook," as she called it. My grandparents had only recently been convinced that their cordless house phone wasn't the same as a cellphone. One day, Pawpaw confidently took the phone around the block on a grocery run. It didn't work. They finally conceded and purchased a cell phone. They kept it off to save minutes by avoiding incoming calls and mainly used it for emergencies. This *was* an emergency. Pawpaw had died.

I texted Damien. He was serving on Deacon duty at church. The girls and I skipped our weekly church ritual. One was sick, and both were napping peacefully in their bedroom. It took a while for him to see my message, too. I weighed it out.

I should pack the kids in the car and go up to Delaware. No, I should wait to hear from someone first. It's not safe to take a sick kid around older people. Okay, I'll wait until I know for sure. I know how Mom is.

We'd been through a similar panic just a few months earlier. In the spring of 2013, I was giving a three-hour lecture one afternoon. My phone was on silent, but my smartwatch kept buzzing. I glanced down to see several calls and missed messages. From the previews, I saw it was my sister Devon repeatedly. It had to be critical. Anxiously, I excused myself from my students and stepped into the hallway to return her call. Devon picked up on the first ring.

"Grandma Michaels died!" Devon blurted out as soon as the call connected. "Mom just texted me, and now she won't answer her phone!"

I released the breath I'd been holding, expecting other tragic news. Annoyance replaced my anxiety.

Grandma Michaels wasn't dead. Well, not our Grandma, anyway. Our Grandma Michaels was our dad's mom, whom we'd known and grown up with our entire lives. However, the woman who had died was *not* our relative. There was no relation.

Sister Michaels, the actual deceased, was the mother of our "Great Uncle," or more aptly, Pawpaw's best friend. My siblings barely knew Sister Michaels. She bore no familial honorifics as "Grandma." I knew her from attending church together in Cincinnati, two hours away from my hometown. Fortunately, I'd heard the sad news of her passing before Devon's dramatic call.

I relayed this information to my sister, but instead of a calming effect, it sent her into a deeper tizzy.

"WHAT?!!! WHY IN THE WORLD WOULD MOM TEXT ME THAT?! I CAN'T BELIEVE HER. SHE KNEW WHAT SHE WAS DOING!" Devon screamed into the receiver.

I closed my eyes and rubbed the edge of my forehead with my free hand. Here we go again. I understood Devon's anger. I didn't have time for it. My class was waiting. I gently interrupted her, told her I'd call her back, and returned to class.

Recalling that story and a sick child had stilled me from automatically jumping on the highway and driving home to find out what happened to Pawpaw. For what felt like an eternity, I paced around my living room, calling every number in my contacts, beginning with area code 740, over and over again. I called my uncle and great-uncle in other states. No one picked up. Finally, after what felt like hours, someone answered.

"Hello."

On the other end of the receiver, I could hear the hustling, bustling, and beeping in the background. She was at the hospital. My heart sank a little.

"Hey, Granny," I opened, trying to be delicate and holding my breath.

"Hey, Bridge," Granny sounded tired but not grief-stricken.

"What's going on?" I held back, not wanting to overwhelm her with a thousand questions.

"Your Dad … I'm sorry, I mean, Pawpaw fainted at church. The doctors are saying that he's dehydrated."

"DEHYDRATED?!?!" I shouted into the receiver. Oops. I caught myself, covering my mouth. I lowered my voice slightly.

"Mom basically said he was DEAD!!!," my filter slipped at the end.

"What? Huh? No. He just needs fluids," Granny sounded as confused as I felt.

"Mom texted me and said he didn't have a pulse!" It was more a question than a statement.

"No, when he passed out, she was having trouble finding his pulse, but when the ambulance came, they found it easily. We're here with him in the emergency room. He's fine."

Anger, relief, fury, dismay, and frustration slurried on my insides. I clenched my lips to keep from saying more. Granny didn't need that. It was a stressful situation. Not life-threatening, but taxing. We got off the phone.

I sat in disbelief. It was as if Mom thought her life was a blockbuster movie. She was the hero in a make-believe Hollywood production. It was as if she'd managed to text me with one hand while doing chest compressions on her dying father with the other. She was the hero, saving her dad from his untimely demise. In reality, it was hot outside, and he fainted. He was transported to the hospital, given fluids, and released the same day.

It was part of her pathology; I'd nearly fallen for it again. I was fed up. As I investigated, I discovered Mom hadn't texted anyone else about this inflammatory misdiagnosis. I was her only target. Everyone else had gotten calls or more detailed texts. Maybe it was because she knew how much my grandparents meant to me. She resented our relationship, and taking it away from me felt good, even for a moment. I don't know her reason, but I was furious. It took me a week before I could talk to her again. I had no idea that it would be the last time.

I went to my Favorites list and hit the icon to speed-dial her number. She picked up on the second ring this time. I went through the usual formalities before diving into the purpose of my call.

"Mom, I wanted to talk to you about your text last week saying that Pawpaw didn't have a pulse. It was terrifying. Then, you didn't answer your phone."

"Well, Bridgette, it was an emergency, and you should feel lucky that I even texted you."

"I hear that it was an emergency, but I'd appreciate it if you wouldn't send me life-or-death texts until you can provide more information."

"Everything isn't about you! You're selfish even to ask me such a thing. You need to be grateful."

"I would be grateful if you didn't send me those types of messages," I responded.

"You're always picking on me. Nothing I do is ever good enough. I'm always the problem. I don't have to take this. Goodbye!" She hung up on me.

I convened and called my people Damien, Devon, and Granny in succession to vent. Mom must've done the same. Over the next three days, I got two calls from outraged relatives. They'd ironed their capes and rushed to Mom's defense.

This wasn't unusual. Mom was skilled in acquiring allies. Her ability to bring third parties into our conflicts, called triangulation, were unmatched. These partners are called enablers or "flying monkeys." I recall learning this term from a colleague and thinking it was the funniest and most appropriate analogy I'd ever heard. Like the Wizard of Oz, these are the people sent out to do the illicit bidding of the narcissist. There are two types: benevolent and malevolent. The benevolent enabler is not consciously trying to cause harm but is wrongly convinced by the narcissist's version of events. They are pulled into rescue mode with strong incentives to take care of the narcissist and stay in their good graces. Then, there is the malevolent enabler. This type of flying monkeys do not mean well. They knowingly participate in the abuse to fulfill their desire for power. They share similar ideas and levels of entitlement as the narcissist and conjointly attack the narcissist's victims.

Mom had a few fixed enablers in her arsenal. No matter what harm Mom causes, they stay on her side. I understand that for them, it is easier to be her friend than her enemy as those are the only two choices in her world. Those who take a more variable approach tend to be the peacekeepers. They may suffer from a need to please her, or they recognize they may need something from her down the line.

Aunt April called me first, a malevolent enabler. April maintained her allies and enemies based on her own needs. Her alliance with my mother was unstable and never lasted long. April took her manipulations a little further than Mom. Mom might pit people against one another behind their backs. April would orchestrate a fight right before your eyes and then sit back with a look of pride and artificial innocence as the drama unfolded. Mom might steal your identity for an electric bill, or your leftover prescription drugs, but April might steal all of the furniture out of your house while you're in jail, or so I've heard.

I listened to April as she tried to back me into agreement.

"Can't you understand that your mom was in the middle of an emergency?" she coaxed.

The problem with that argument was that Mom knew Pawpaw had a pulse. He was already in the ambulance when she texted me. She also had time to go home and change clothes before driving to the hospital, but she didn't answer my calls. I held my ground.

April was only a few years older than me. I was always a little afraid of her when we were children; most people were. She knew it. I'd seen her fight near-grown men and shrink full-grown adults with her fierce words. April believed that she could outwit anyone. She was smart and usually could. By now, she'd lived away from the family for some years. I'd grown up and was no longer the passive, naive teen she was used to. I saw through her and her maneuvers. She seemed to sense that she'd met her match on a cognitive level. Never to be bested, she resorted back to a primal base, aggression.

"Look, you're only the granddaughter! You don't have a right to know anything. You better stay in your lane," she warned angrily.

I didn't argue or escalate. It was pointless. It didn't matter. I *did* have a right to be informed about what happened with my grandparents. I was one of the executors of their estates. My grandparents' binding legal decision had disrupted the imaginary familial hierarchy. I was one of the trusted ones. Trusted with information. Relied on to carry out their wishes regardless of who disagreed. All of the hostile posturing only made my aunt feel better. It took nothing from me to let her have it.

The next call, though, surprised me. It was my brother, Tony. He never calls me, ever. We've never really had direct problems and used to be close as teens. We're good when we see each other with hugs and hellos. We're fine, not close.

He, too, had gotten a version of events from Mom that made it seem like I was ungrateful and bullying Mom about her text. Knowing Mom, Tony seemed quickly amenable to my account and the true nature of my request for her not to text me that type of information. He replied, "Oh." I was momentarily relieved, but it passed too soon.

"I have another bone to pick with you. You and Devon were wrong for making fun of Mom for wearing scrubs to the hospital!"

The day Pawpaw fainted, instead of going straight to the hospital, Mom had gone home to change into a pair of scrubs. Yes, Devon, I, and most of the family got annoyed at Mom's self-aggrandizing nursing performance in any healthcare situation. She hadn't worked as a medical assistant in nearly 20 years. That didn't stop her from dressing the part, speaking on behalf of the patient, seeking attention for her feigned ailments over the actual patient, and pushing her way into exam and surgical rooms without patient consent. It was frustrating when it happened, but this case had a problem.

I have no idea what my mom wore or didn't wear. I don't know what she did or didn't do at the hospital that day. I can assume from past behavior, but I don't know. I don't have a clue because I wasn't there; Devon wasn't there. We lived 2- and 24-hours away, respectively, at the time. Somehow, Mom had convinced Tony that we'd come together to make fun of Mom's scrubs across all that distance.

It was one thing for Mom to lie on me, been there, done that, got the T-shirt, but I was deeply wounded that reality and the apparent truth hadn't countered the false narrative. I felt it deep in my soul. That realization that there was nothing I could do to protect myself from her. It broke something new in me.

I screamed in raw emotional pain at Tony, "DID *YOU* EVEN SEE ME THERE?"

It wasn't the worst lie Mom had ever told on me. It wasn't the most despicable thing she ever had or would say about me. It wasn't the evilest thing she could do to me in the world. But, it was the *last*.

I cried one last good cry, a cry of grief. I grieved the loss of a mother I never had and would never be. The seasons of denial, anger, bargaining, depression, acceptance ended.[3] I forgave her eventually but I had to love her from afar. It was the only way to honor my mother.

As I dried my tears, the eeriest calm washed over me, a sense of peace. I didn't call Mom to share my decision. There was nothing to explain or discuss. I recognize that leaving a narcissist launches an onslaught of predictable manipulation and attacks.[4, 5] She will cry and cuss you. She will badmouth and blame you. She will vow to do better and promise to change in attempts to win you back, a strategy called hoovering. She won't change. They can't change. Mom may have never appreciated the immediate cause of my departure, but on some level she knew what she'd done. The final straw was of no consequence.

I went no contact with Mom. It wasn't easy. I stopped answering her calls and texts. I eventually had to block her number and screen my calls. She tried to reach me on other numbers. I hung up immediately or ignore the texts. I didn't open or acknowledge her emails or letters. She tried to reach out on social media, and I deleted and blocked her. I asked others to protect my privacy and not share my personal information with her. It was difficult for some, especially Granny, who felt caught in the middle. I moved to a new house and hoped that would create more distance. Mom didn't have my address. Granny resisted giving it to her directly but let her copy it off some mail I'd sent to the house. Mom sent something to my daughters. I sent it back.

Yes, my no-contact position extended to my children. As their mother, I must protect them from poor judgment, manipulation, drug use, and emotional and physical abuse. Mom had finagled a disability check that she supplemented with babysitting jobs. Stories of my mother smoking in front of children or disoriented from prescription narcotics while watching children continued to leak through the family. Her brother allegedly nearly came to blows with her because she spanked his five-month-old son for "not sitting still" during a diaper change. She was once babysitting the child of a cousin on my dad's side of the family. The girl is the victim of incest at the hands of another child in Mom's care. She whipped both children, reasoning that the young girl "let it happen." Devon lost it on Mom after she struck my oldest nephew with a karate staff. That was Devon's last-straw moment. After being a teenage mother, she now found herself in a supportive and loving relationship with Charles, whom she eventually married. She no longer had to subject her children to Mom's dysfunction.

It was these kinds of stories that solidified my decision. I would unapologetically shelter my children like few adults did for me as a child. If my girls decide to have a relationship with their grandmother when they are adults, it's up to them. For now, my intent is not to control or convince them of the dangers of their grandmother but to protect them.

I have to have occasional contact with my mother at family functions, where I try to stay on my side of the boxing ring. Sometimes, she'll push the issue, come close, or force me into a hug. I always speak with the obligatory "hello" and promptly return to my corner, only to hear stories later that I "attacked" her. To a narcissist, being ignored probably does feel like an emotional assault, but Mom's interpretation was no longer my concern. I was in balance. She could not shake me.

Mom will use my response to her actions, boundaries, as a way to reinforce and justify her perceived victimhood. In time, she'll pursue new persuasive tactics. She'll likely claim she's going to therapy, giving hope to others of the possibility of change, but really seeking validation for her actions and attempting to undermine my professional expertise.[6] She might take to social media to find support among other alienated parents. Maybe she'll turn her journals into a counter-argumentative book. She may even engage in self-harm to firmly establish herself as the aggrieved. I'd hate for that to happen but it's a harsh reality I must acknowledge. However, all that I wish for her is the light and love she could not give her children.

This time, no amount of cultural, religious, or family pressure tempted me to give in. Our relationship was over. I was done. Guilt free. That last thin artery tethering our lives together was finally severed. Our relationship flatlined.

No pulse.

References

1. Centers for Disease Control and Prevention (CDC). (n.d.). *Fast facts: Preventing adverse childhood experiences.* https://www.cdc.gov/violenceprevention/aces/fastfact.html

2. National Academies of Sciences, Engineering, and Medicine (2016). *Parenting Matters: Supporting Parents of Children Ages 0–8.* Washington, DC: The National Academies Press. https://doi.org/10.17226/21868

3. Kübler-Ross, E. (1970). *On death and dying.* Macmillan.

4. Grande, D. (2023). *Going no contact with a narcissist: Everything you need to know. Choosing therapy.* https://www.choosingtherapy.com/no-contact-with-a-narcissist/#:~:text=Going%20no%20contact%20often%20negatively,collapse%2C%20depression%2C%20or%20anger.

5. Rosenberg, R. (2022). *When you unmask a covert narcissist, RUN, but quietly! medium.* http://www.https://medium.com/@Ross-Rosenberg/when-you-unmask-a-covert-narcissist-run-but-quietly

6. Arabi, S. (2017, August 14). *5 Ways pathologically envious narcissists undermine your success. PsychCentral.* https://psychcentral.com/blog/recovering-narcissist/2017/08/5-ways-pathologically-envious-narcissists-undermine-your-success#1

CHAPTER 15

"You Can't Spell Families Without Lies"[1]

Adverse Childhood Experiences and Religion

For many survivors of ACEs, faith can be a powerful source of healing, offering community, purpose, and hope. Religious beliefs and practices can foster resilience, providing a framework for meaning-making and emotional regulation.[2] However, faith can also be misused—weaponized by abusers to justify harm, silence victims, or demand unquestioning obedience.[3]

"BRIDGE, CAN I ask you something and you promise not to get mad?"

The monitor above Granny's head beeped. It and the television across the room were the only things illuminating the sterile hospital room. By now, I knew all the nurses by name and was growing desensitized to the smell of human degeneration. Family and friends had retired for the day, and Granny and I settled into our evening routine, hand-holding and watching home design shows. On the nights Granny could speak; she'd pass down her matriarchal wisdom and family secrets.

"So-and-so is just young and needs to mature. So-and-so needs a little extra love and attention. So-and-so shouldn't get married. So-and-so has a secret to tell all of you."

The first "so-and-so" was my age and the last has never told their secret. Accepting these insights felt like a push into her role as the family matriarch, a position I hadn't applied for and didn't want. I wasn't built for it. I was no "Granny" with immeasurable wisdom, high naiveté, and an infinite capacity for forgiveness. I'm highly sensitive to manipulation. I value personal accountability. And, my version of forgiveness differed from hers.

"Yes, Granny. I'll try not to get upset."

I held my breath, wondering what she was going to say next.

"First, I love you so much," Granny shared.

I believed her. But I still noticed that she'd primed my emotional response by asking me not to get angry before making her request. Now, she was trying to further disarm me with love. I'm not going to lie; given the circumstances, it worked.

"Second, I just don't understand why you can't forgive your mother."

The weight of her request echoed off the walls of her hospice room where she'd been transferred three days prior. This was her dying wish: forgiveness between mother and daughter. I wondered if she too had forgiven her daughter for the latest wounds she'd inflicted. I knew I wasn't ready.

"I have forgiven her for the past," I offered Granny, trying to sound nonchalant.

It felt true, mostly. I wasn't hanging onto the past; however, I was furious with Mom in the present. Granny didn't need to hear that right now, though.

"You don't talk to her," Granny countered.

Granny believed in a kind of forgiveness that was rapid and reengaging. She seemed to have an uncanny ability to sustain a hurt and brush it off like scrambled eggs on a Teflon-coated skillet. It was the only evidence of Godly forgiveness, no matter the circumstance. She was more of a spiritual heavyweight than I was, and for a long time, I thought she was right. For my salvation, I believed I had to engage with my mother. I wrestled with this idea until I finally felt settled in my spirit in recent years.

I knew forgiveness was a cognitive process, a way of thinking. It's necessary for our healing. It releases us from the position of victim and transforms us into survivors. It is empowering. But forgiveness does not mean the person will change, nor does it mean that it's healthy to remain in a relationship with an abusive person.[4–6] Period.

I steadied myself and responded.

"Granny, I don't have to be in contact with Mom to forgive her. Not being around her helps me stay in a forgiving place."

Granny continued as if I hadn't spoken.

"When I was an adult, my mom punched me in the face and dragged me down the stairs by my hair, and I still forgave her."

I wondered if Granny understood the full extent of her comparison. Was the physical abuse I endured somehow acceptable because I had been a child? Was it better because I was habitually slapped rather than punched? Was it more tolerable that my blood spilled from welts delivered via the extension cord rather than a fist? Did Mom's emotional and psychological abuse and neglect not count? Did our victimization at the hands of Mom's sexual predator partners mean nothing?

The room was quiet as we both likely reflected on our abusive mothers.

I'd grown so much in the four years since I stopped engaging with Mom. I was grateful for the 3G's (Granny, God, and graduate school) that had each played a role in the early phases of my adverse childhood experiences (ACEs) recovery. Somewhere along the way, though, I learned to trust myself too. My view mattered. I could see clearly. I could choose for myself. It wasn't for Granny to validate. It wasn't a salvation issue. It wasn't for anyone else to agree. And it was psychologically healthy. It was right for me when I decided that I had had enough. I couldn't make Granny a false promise.

"I'm so sorry that happened to you, Granny. You didn't deserve for your mom to do that. No one does. I'm sorry you felt you had to accept that. I would not have."

It broke my heart that, at 80 years old, Granny had never been free from the weight of an abusive mother and that she carried that burden almost as a point of pride. Her mother had been dead since before I was born, yet Granny continued to defend her honor. Her major act of resistance was to do the opposite type of mothering with her children. It was the best Granny could do, but the results were mixed. Some of her children regressed, and others strived to do better. As a psychologist, I felt I had even more tools to do more earlier on in my life. I, too, was doing the best I could with what I knew.

"Well, we were saying how you treat your patients better than you treat your own mother. I just don't understand it," Granny posed.

I was caught off guard. The "we," most likely, were Granny and Mom. Most of the family had little to do with Mom by now, and Pawpaw rarely engaged in these debates. No matter how much I tried to escape the Bermuda Triangle between Granny, Mom, and me, I was always a central figure.

"I see you all have been practicing your arguments," a short laugh escaped before I could catch it. I meant no disrespect.

"Most of my patients acknowledge that there is a problem and want to get help. I'm also not usually the target of my patients' pathologies."

Granny wasn't making it easy, asking sobering end-of-life questions and coming at me from new angles. Two days earlier, she'd also questioned me about Mom. I almost fumbled the answers then, too.

"Has Debra come to see me, and I just can't remember?" Granny had asked somberly one night.

It wasn't a real question. Granny's health was failing, but her memory was intact. Mom hadn't been back to see her in the weeks since her initial hospitalization. Mom had even ignored Granny's distress calls five days before her hospital admission.

Granny had been uncertain whether her pain and diminished appetite warranted a trip to an expensive emergency room (ER). She'd called her oldest daughter, Debra, the "nurse," daily, only for her calls to be ignored or sent to voicemail. I offered to remove the financial barrier and pay the hospital copay as an incentive. Let a licensed healthcare provider determine if it was an emergency. It would give us all peace of mind, which I needed, especially because I was leaving on a five-day family cruise the next day and would have intermittent mobile service.

The vacation was bittersweet. The cruise line customer service and experience was phenomenal, but I was distracted. Granny had been admitted to the hospital from the ER, and I was getting irregular updates. They knew she was sick but didn't know why. She'd been through several scans and tests, but we had no answers.

The day after our ship docked stateside and before our lost luggage ever arrived, I packed up the girls in the car and drove to see Granny an hour and a half away. Out of concern, Uncle Brian was also visiting from Washington, DC. He and Pawpaw were sitting by Granny's bedside. The oncologist, a middle-aged Black man, came into the room to tell us the results of Granny's scans. He asked if it would be okay if my daughters went into the hallway to draw with one of the nurses. I initially resisted not wanting to leave my children with a stranger, but the look on his face told me the news was grave. I relented.

Adenocarcinoma, bile duct cancer, was the diagnosis. It had likely lingered and spread since Granny's bout with gallbladder cancer a few years prior. The intermittent follow-up MRIs hadn't caught it. Now, it was too late. Surgery was too risky, and Granny was too frail.

"What's the prognosis?" I choked out barely above a whisper.

"Not good. At this rate, she's looking at 2–3 months."

The doctor offered some hope, "maybes" for surgery "if" she got stronger. I could feel his inauthenticity. It was his way of silver-lining the dark cloud that had cast over the room before making his hasty escape.

We all wanted to stay with Granny, but none of us could. I had the girls. Uncle Brian had to take Pawpaw home for kidney dialysis. Out of options, Pawpaw relented and asked Mom to come and stay.

"She's not in our phone directory. She took the phone and deleted her number without telling us a few weeks ago. I have to scroll through the call list whenever I need to find her," Pawpaw said.

I held my tongue. Pawpaw rubbed his forehead, eyes closed as he dialed Mom's number. This time, she answered.

"Debra, I need you to come and stay at the hospital with your mother tonight."

"I can't because I'm not feeling well. I'm sick," Mom claimed.

"It's really important, and I need you to come," Pawpaw pleaded.

"What's this about? I saw Brian's text about a family call tonight."

We'd set up a conference call and sent out a message to get the family on one accord with information. The news would be draining, and we didn't want to repeat ourselves repeatedly or have the message get lost on the gossip vine. Some were resentful that the invite list extended beyond Granny's children. Others were mad that they didn't receive the message on their disconnected phone numbers. Mom flat-out refused to join. I was too exhausted from the news of Granny's health to worry about their gripes.

"I'm not getting on the call for them to gang up on me," Mom raged.

"It's not about YOU. Just be quiet, get on the call, and get here after!" Pawpaw demanded of his oldest child.

In his old age, he rarely yelled, so when he did, we immediately complied. Mom obeyed. It would take him using the same approach weeks later to get her to return.

Meanwhile, the family convened from the four corners of the United States to set up camp and a 24-hour vigil over Granny. During the day, 10–12 visitors rotated in from the waiting room. At night, Devon and I mostly alternated shifts. Mom lived 20 minutes away and was nowhere to be found. No visits, no overnights for weeks.

Mom's siblings called her and begged her to visit her mother. She ran through her usual excuses, poor health, and blaming others. Mom said she was going through a breast cancer scare. It turned out she'd long known that she was in the clear. A church elder reached out to her inquiring about her absence. She told him Devon and I were "abusive" when she came to the hospital. He shared this with us almost as if to ask us to be nicer to Mom the next time she came. When was the first time she'd come? We reminded him that she'd never been there with my sister and me. We'd seen him, the elder frequently, never Mom.

Granny was getting antsy and wanted answers. There was an overlay of sadness in her inquisitions. *Where is my daughter?*

Professionally, I knew this was a standard question at Granny's developmental stage. She wanted to leave the world fulfilled, knowing that she'd left a strong, positive family legacy and that she'd been a good mother overall. In psychology, we call this phase integrity versus despair. This assessment and summary of one's life is often triggered by significant shifts such as retirement, loss of a spouse, or terminal illness. Mom's absence likely ignited doubt about Granny's long-term contributions to her family and caused feelings of sadness and regret that she wanted to resolve.

I won't romanticize her life completely. Granny could be naggy, needy, and neurotic at times. She believed sincerely in social dangers—dancing, dishonesty, and drinking—all equal paths to damnation. She set the bar high, too high for us to reach. Some gave up, and some of us kept trying, but Granny was there for us through it all. Likely, in Granny's mind, Mom's absence was a sign that she'd failed her mission. That she'd somehow done irreparable damage to one of her children. If Granny blamed herself, I couldn't let her leave the world believing that fallacy.

"Uh, I'm not here all of the time. Sometimes, I take a break to rest at the hotel. I might've missed her or something. I'm not sure."

I hoped Granny would buy my explanation. I avoided her full, all-knowing gaze. Did she buy it? I'm uncertain whether she caught onto my tactics, but she didn't follow up. I released a breath I didn't realize I was holding. I felt proud of my creativity and that I hadn't raised anything negative despite my feelings about Mom's desertion.

At Pawpaw's command, Mom eventually obliged. Devon and I were forced to abandon our post at Granny's bedside for the night. We were exhausted but reluctant to leave the hospital. Mom would throw a wrench in our routine.

I returned as soon as I woke, less than 12 hours later. The morning nurse, Kim, stopped me in the hallway before I got to Granny's room.

"Who is that lady in there? She had two of my nurses written up last night."

"Yeah, that's my mom, Granny's oldest daughter. I'm so sorry. I rescind any complaints made about your staff. You all have been doing a remarkable job."

Mom had complained about the nursing staff, saying that Granny hadn't been bathed in days. First, how would she know? Second, untrue. Devon and I bathed Granny daily. Mom also filed a complaint that Granny had a bed sore the "size of a football" on her back. It was about the size of a quarter, and the wound care team had already been dressing it. Mom had tossed out an industrial air fresher we'd been using to mask the smell in the room, saying it was "disrespectful." Granny had expressed embarrassment about the odor wafting from her colostomy bag. We were doing our best to help offset it.

In one night, Mom had physically taken over the hospital room. It was her routine of centering herself in any situation. The seats and sofa were filled with bags, clothes, blankets, pillows, crocheting, and snacks. We had to move her stuff out of the way for anyone to sit. She later told people we "threw [her] bags on the floor."

For Granny's sake, I didn't complain. This time with her oldest daughter was for her. So, we worked around Mom that morning, reestablishing our disrupted care system. We were only a few hours into our efforts when my Aunt April showed me a series of text messages from Mom.

"Bridgette can't handle this," one read.

"She's been in and out of the room all day!" another text said.

But I had been handling it—for two weeks. I didn't bite. Mom's criticisms didn't matter. My aunt's messiness in sharing the texts didn't either. She'd actually defended me, questioning my mother about her absence, but I wasn't interested in faux and temporary alliances either. The only person who mattered was Granny.

The experience did give me more insight into the depth of Mom's narcissism. I'd allowed myself to believe that the prospect of her mother's death would override her pathological self-centeredness and irrational thinking. I'd fallen into the trap again, only to be reminded that people with personality disorders do not change. I had to stop expecting it. This insight sent me to a new level of doneness, permanently sealing the casket of our relationship. Mom was dead to me. Meanwhile, Granny was dying.

So, I responded when Granny asked me on her penultimate day of life why I couldn't forgive my mother.

"Granny, you know I love you too, and you know I'd do *anything* for you," I maneuvered, borrowing her tactics. I squeezed her warm hand for emphasis.

"I wish I could tell you I could go back, but I honestly can't. My life has been much more peaceful and emotionally healthier all these years without her. I won't give that up," I pleaded.

My gut sat unwavering—not resistant, but resolved. I would no longer play the role of an impostor. I'd relinquished familial and societal expectations of compliance and not succumbed to guilt under the worst pressure imaginable. I'd allowed myself to share my genuine beliefs and had spoken in my true voice. I was living authentically and unapologetically. As I stood firm at Granny's hospital bedside, a deep realization dawned on me—my impostorism had healed.

This is how I honored Granny's profound legacy. She hadn't been able to break *all* of the generational curses, but she'd shattered many. She'd accomplished that with a 10th-grade education, religion, and sheer will. I'd built on what she started, eradicating the cancerous recurrence caused by my mother in between generations and creating a liberated path for our descendents.

My heart skipped with joy at the realization—but Granny didn't miss a beat.

"Well, in Exodus 20:12, the Bible says … ," she said, reverting to her biblical arguments. I'd grown used to it. All I could do was smile.

Granny ended her sermonette and the night saying her prayers aloud, closing by asking God to soften my heart. I think He only heard the "heart" part because instead of softening, a piece would be broken.

***

Two days later, Devon and I returned to Granny's hospital room early on an unseasonably warm Wednesday morning in January. We walked side by side, winding through the now-familiar building. They'd finally figured out a way for Pawpaw to stay overnight, and he'd been permitted to do his mobile kidney dialysis onsite. It'd seemed to pain him every day when he left his wife's side for dinner and dialysis, leaving one of his granddaughters to hold vigil instead of doing it himself.

When Devon and I entered the room, Granny whipped her head toward us.

HELP!

Granny's eyes pleaded silently at me as she gripped the crisp, white hospital sheets in her right hand and Pawpaw's dark, withering hand with her left.

Pawpaw was using his free hand to pat the top of Granny's thin, jet-black hair. It was meant to be comforting, but I knew it annoyed her. I'd twice overheard her asking him to stop "petting her like a dog" since she'd been admitted to the hospital.

He continued stroking her hair like a man who'd operated machines his whole life. I loved him for trying. Out of respect, I couldn't redirect him. She was *his* wife.

Granny turned her head between Pawpaw and me as if to say, "I'm trying to tell him," as she strained for air.

I rushed out of the room to find Sarah, the hospice nurse, a tall, curly-haired blonde woman who had been our tour guide through death and dying. She returned to the room with me and checked Granny's breathing with a stethoscope. She looked into my eyes and gave me the slightest nod. It was time.

We quickly made urgent calls to family before resuming our posts, Pawpaw on Granny's left and Devon and I on her right. We sat in silence, listening to Granny's breaths. Trying to stay present, I counted them.

… One one thousand, two one thousand, three one thousand, four one thousand, five one thousand. A single breath.

… One one thousand, two one thousand, three one thousand, four one thousand, five one thousand, six one thousand. *Breath.*

… One one thousand, two one thousand, three one thousand, four one thousand, five one thousand, sixxxx one thousand, sevennnnn one thousand, eeeeeight one thousand. *Breath.*

I was breathing with Granny and starting to feel aches in my lungs as the time stretched too long between her momentary gasps for air.

Six seconds.
Nine seconds.
Eight seconds.
Twelve seconds.

Every time Granny inhaled, the relief was fleeting, and I started counting again.

After about 30 minutes, my slow count finally reached 20; I couldn't hold my breath any longer. I let out a pained breath. Granny didn't.

Moments passed, and no one spoke up. It didn't feel like it was my place to call her death, so we continued sitting in silence. It felt like an hour, but it was probably four minutes before Pawpaw stood up from his chair shakily.

"Welp, that's it," was all he could manage.

Though nothing fell to his cheeks, his eyes were red and rimmed wet. It was the closest I'd ever seen him to tears. He kissed Granny's temple and stood quietly by her side before slumping into his seat in a daze that would last for months.

I closed my eyes to the hot tears and took in slow, deep breaths for a long time until my body calmed. Devon and I clung to Granny for hours, knowing it would be the last time she'd comfort us.

Death and dying were nothing like I envisioned. Inexperience convinced me I'd be afraid, but it wasn't scary. Melancholy at times, but in a way, it was also beautiful, especially our routine—sponging, lotioning, fluffing, shifting, one leg left uncovered to breathe. Granny would choose her perfume and try to eat on our behalf. We'd greet visitors, tell jokes, pray, retell family stories, and guide excessively bereaved guests to the lobby. It was always the ones who bore no relation that seemed to be doing the most. In her death, we wanted Granny to feel love, joy, and peace, the things she'd tried to give us in life. Even in death, she tried to care for us by putting on a brave front. We were doing the same for her.

That time caring for her was a small repayment for all she'd done for me. I owed her so much more. She saved my life by letting me move in with them. I wouldn't be the woman I am today without her. It dawned on me at that moment that *she* was my mother. She'd given me what a mother was supposed to and what my mother could not. I'd already let go of my biological mother, so I felt motherless when Granny passed.

There was a strange sense of isolation and of being alone in this world. Nothing ahead of me, looking out and warning me about life's unknown dangers. No one else could love me and understand me the way Granny had. I felt lost for a moment, but in the following months, I began to reflect on the outpouring of love I received when I lost Granny. The women who held things down for me at work, the friends who cooked us meals, the family friends who handled her cremation free of charge, and the ones who reminded me that tears were a sign that I had loved. Mothering doesn't only come from the ones who birth you. These women were my "othermothers."

World-renowned sociologist Dr. Patricia Hill Collins describes "othermothers" as nonbiological mothers who fulfill the emotional, psychological, and educational needs of those in their extended families, educational institutions, and communities. They achieve this through caring, guiding, and teaching those around them. They step in to fill the gaps and can help alleviate some of the stressors found in mother–daughter relationships. These women include older siblings, aunts and "aunties," neighbors, teachers, mentors, and friends. I realized that I had countless othermothers, and cumulatively, they and others have sustained me in Granny's absence and beyond. The mothering I needed wasn't encompassed all in one person but was spread out among these women. As I recognized how they'd poured into me, I realized that I'd become an othermother somewhere along the way, too.

As much as I resisted stepping into the official role of family matriarch, I was mothering in all facets of my life. My relatives come to me for academic, financial, and relationship advice. I mentor students who are primarily women of color and the first in their families to attend college and graduate school. My friends and colleagues often seek me out for my views and perspectives. I teach and volunteer in churches, community service agencies, and at my children's schools to help uplift those around me. I am a therapist. This is me being a matriarch, not just for my children, but for those around me in my community, in my culture.

This role differs from what I envisioned when Granny sought to bestow this inheritance upon me. I rejected it because I believed I had to do it "her way," and I knew I'd fail. I'm not her. I could never be. I was me. Over the decades, I've grown comfortable with who I am and realized I have something valuable to contribute to those around me, even if it is in a different way.

***

Avery, a 27-year-old unemployed Jamaican mother of one, currently separated, sought therapy with a history of unexplained mood swings and a traumatic childhood punctuated by ACEs. Her mother, who grappled with untreated mental illness, an undiagnosed personality disorder, and addiction, abandoned her when she was just

11 years old, leaving Avery in the care of her father and an emotionally abusive stepmother in the United States. Tragically, her mother took her own life one year before Avery began therapy, a rare act in Caribbean culture.

Religion served as a dual-edged sword in Avery's life. While it provided her with support and inner strength, it also inadvertently reinforced the acceptance of parental abuse. She was frequently discouraged from discussing her ACEs under the guise of demonstrating "respect" and "gratitude" toward her biological parents and stepmother. This pressure intensified after her mother's passing as she looked to conceptualize her childhood abuse and was advised by some of her biological and church family members not to "speak ill of the dead."

Avery's strong spiritual and cultural beliefs significantly influenced her initial resistance to a referral for psychiatric medication. In addition, she'd never sought prior psychotherapy and had solely received pastoral counseling for support and spiritual guidance, leaving her mental illness untreated. Consequently, her mood swings and trauma responses profoundly affected her daily functioning and her ability to maintain healthy interpersonal relationships. At the time, she was unemployed, grappling with a strained relationship with her spouse and experiencing difficulties in her extended family connections.

Avery was diagnosed with bipolar disorder, which manifested through intermittent episodes of depression and manic states. She also displayed symptoms of complex trauma, which led to various behavioral, emotional, and interpersonal challenges. These difficulties included impulsivity, episodes of rage, and a pronounced struggle to form secure attachments with others. Moreover, Avery harbored a deeply ingrained belief that she was undeserving of love and respect, a negative self-perception rooted in her traumatic upbringing. Furthermore, the grief over her mother's death proved to be an incredibly complex and conflicted process for Avery. She vacillated between feelings of anger, guilt, and unresolved grief, making it difficult for her to process her emotions and mourn her mother's passing properly.

We collaborated to establish a comprehensive treatment plan for Avery primarily centered around cognitive behavioral therapy (CBT) techniques for ACEs survivors.[7] This approach aimed to address her maladaptive thoughts, feelings, and behaviors while also helping her recover from the effects of parental narcissistic abuse. Our treatment plan was designed to reframe her negative beliefs, regulate her emotions, develop healthier coping strategies, and foster resilience. I encouraged Avery to seek pastoral counseling to clarify her church's position on mental illness and medicinal interventions. To complement the primary treatment approaches, we also incorporated Dr. Karyl McBride's book, *Will I Ever Be Good Enough?: Healing the Daughters of Narcissistic Mothers*. Avery found the tools in this book to be particularly resonant and helpful in her recovery.

One tool, doll therapy, was an unconventional component of her rehabilitation. Avery bought a doll that resembled herself and used it to engage in soothing and restorative play.[8] She engaged in careful grooming, which served as a countermeasure to the neglect she experienced as a child. Additionally, Avery employed the doll to practice positive affirmations to counteract the verbal abuse she had endured. She reported that these interactions with the doll and journaling homework to document her experiences were instrumental in her growth.

Doll therapy provided Avery with a safe space to practice self-compassion and heightened self-awareness. It allowed her to acknowledge the maternal abuse she had endured without guilt openly. She could grieve the mother she had rather than an idealized version.

In consultation with her pastor,[9] Avery gradually recognized the advantages of mood-regulating medications and, under her psychiatrist's guidance, began a prescription of lithium. In conjunction with her therapy sessions, she gained better control over her mood swings, leading to a noticeable reduction in the frequency and intensity of her manic and depressive episodes. Avery acquired the ability to identify her trauma triggers and learned how to manage them through breathing and relaxation techniques. These therapeutic interventions significantly enhanced her familial and marital relationships, bolstered her self-esteem, allowed her to move through her grief, and improved her sense of personal competence.

Eventually, Avery relocated and continued her therapy with another practitioner. For the first year she checked in with me to share her ongoing progress. Most recently, she experienced the joy of expanding her family with another child and ventured into entrepreneurship.

Avery could have continued living in anger and burning bridges along the way. She could have colluded with family and religious figures in minimizing her abuse. She could have passed her trauma down to her kids. Instead, she turned and faced it. She learned to regulate her emotions and communicate her needs. With this progress, she may still never fully regain what was lost in her childhood. All we can hope for is continued growth.

***

Back in that moment when my mother told me she didn't think I'd be any good at helping people as a psychologist, I can now say with certainty—she was wrong. This work has not been in vain. At the very least, it has helped me heal, making space for one less traumatized person in the world. At its mid-point, perhaps a client or a reader will see themselves in these stories I've shared, feel less alone, and continue the difficult work of healing. At its best, it might inspire us to take collective action—protecting children from ACEs and preventing the devastating physical and mental health outcomes they bring.

Whether child or adult, survivors deserve to feel seen, safe, and supported. No one should have to face the weight of their childhood alone. Together, we can help them move from surviving to truly living.

References

1. Gordon, S. (2008). Four christmases [Film]. New Line Cinema, Spyglass Entertainment and Warner Bros.

2. Freeny, J., Peskin, M., Schick, V., Cuccaro, P., Addy, R., Morgan, R., . . . Johnson-Baker, K. (2021). Adverse childhood experiences, depression, resilience, & spirituality in African-American adolescents. *Journal of Child & Adolescent Trauma*, *14*(2), 209–221. https://doi.org/10.1007/s40653-020-00335-91

3. Ellis, H. M., Hook, J. N., Zuniga, S., Hodge, A. S., Ford, K. M., Davis, D. E., & Van Tongeren, D. R. (2022). Religious/spiritual abuse and trauma: A systematic review of the empirical literature. *Spirituality in Clinical Practice*, *9*, 213–231.

4. Lamb, S. (2005). Forgiveness therapy: The context and conflict. *Journal of Theoretical and Philosophical Psychology*, *25*(1), 61–80.

5. McNulty, J. K., & Russell, V. M. (2016). Forgive and forget, or forgive and regret? Whether forgiveness leads to less or more offending depends on offender agreeableness. *Personality & social psychology bulletin*, *42*(5), 616–631. https://doi.org/10.1177/0146167216637841

6. Alfano, M., & Norlock, K. J. (2017). The challenges of forgiveness in context: Introduction to the moral psychology of forgiveness. In *The moral psychology of forgiveness*. Rowman & Littlefield International.

7. Korotana, L. M., Dobson, K. S., Pusch, D., & Josephson, T. (2016). A review of primary care interventions to improve health outcomes in adult survivors of adverse childhood experiences. *Clinical psychology review*, *46*, 59–90. https://doi.org/10.1016/j.cpr.2016.04.007

8. McBride, K. (2008). *Will I ever be good enough?: Healing the daughters of narcissistic mothers*. Simon and Schuster.

9. Best, M. C., Washington, J., Jones, K., Brunker, M., & Kearney, M. (2024). Measuring the impact of a pastoral care intervention to increase referrals and improve the quality of chaplain documentation in patient records. *Journal of Health Care Chaplaincy*, *31*(2), 1–14.

CHAPTER 16

This Girl Is on Fire

Psychological Minimization

Minimization is a psychological defense mechanism used by abusers and the abused.[1-3] *It involves downplaying the severity of the abuse often to avoid accountability or as a coping mechanism to avoid feelings of shame. It can be conscious or an unconscious invisible weight.*

IT'S CLOUDY TODAY. It must be getting ready to rain. I love listening to the rain. It's so relaxing.

My subconscious mind waited for the inevitable pitter-patter of raindrops. They never came.

Hmm, it's quiet outside too. That's nice. So peaceful.

The silence of my house made sense. It was summer, and my girls were back East visiting my in-laws. We were three months into the COVID-19 lockdown, and the already outdoorsy Californians had taken it to another level, running, biking, and hiking. That day, I didn't hear any balls bouncing, people learning and failing to rollerblade, or families gliding past on their new bikes. It was still. Too still.

It's getting late. I should eat today.

I'd been feverishly typing up stories from my journal for this book well into the afternoon. Hunger pangs pulled me from my trance. I grabbed my purse and headed down to the garage. I put on my new polarized sunglasses to prevent myself from getting a migraine and pressed the button on the preset garage opener. Sunlight didn't come rushing into the dark space like usual. I lifted my glasses, confused.

Wow, it's incredibly cloudy today. It's going to pour. That orange glow behind the clouds is stunning though. It looks kinda like sunset but it's only 2 o'clock.

(dis)Honor Thy Mother: Daughterhood, Dysfunction and Deliverance, First Edition. Bridgette Peteet.

I've never seen an Ohio sky look like that. California had so many hidden beauties. I pulled off and around the corner to the subdivision mailboxes. I got out and noticed delicate white flakes billowing through the air. I smiled at the familiar sight: snow. Something seemed off, though. I mentally scanned my skin thermoreceptors. It was too warm. I'd been doing this mental skin check every time a Californian said it was "cold." I never felt it; usually, it was 68° when they made this assessment. They assured me that I'd adapt eventually. I knew snow air though and it wasn't nearly chilly enough for snowfall.

Maybe the snow drifted through the clouds from the nearby mountains. Cool.

I looked north toward Mt. Baldy, but the summits were shrouded in a thick haze. I'd finally found a love for the snow in those peaks. I could admire the captivating beauty of the ice while sitting warmly in the tepid temperatures below.

Whimsically, I caught a flake midair, cupping it in my hand. A momentary childhood joy came over me. I looked down, expecting to catch a quick glimpse of an intricate crystal star before it melted away. Nothing happened. I did a double take at the tiny gray curl that hadn't liquified in the heat of my palm. *What was this?* It was familiar and yet strange. Like when we'd camp, the wind would blow smoke and ash from the fire pit.

ASH!?!?!? This is a wildfire! I'm in the middle of a forest fire. OK, not the center, but close enough.

I flung the residue to the ground and looked around feverishly to see how other people acted in this apparent wildfire emergency. Smoky the Bear had been telling us how to prevent a forest fire throughout my childhood, but he'd said nothing about what to do once one starts.

Is the fire nearby? Am I allowed to be outside? Should I be breathing this air? Do I need a mask? Do I need to take cover?

I looked to other humans for guidance, scanning my surroundings and snapping mental polaroid photos.

A car driving residential speeds down the street.

A woman casually walking her caramel multipoo on the grassy knoll between the townhouses.

The still shots began to converge into a slow-moving film again. No one seemed to be evacuating or scrambling to safety. My parasympathetic nervous system began to pump the breaks on my fight-or-flight response.

Ok. Got it. It's NOT an emergency. I was safe.

My new California friends got a kick out of this story and others as we adjusted to life in the West. Nature is different out here. Earthquakes weren't always major catastrophes like on television. You might feel one quarterly and still aren't sure if it was just a large truck that drove past until you Google it.

My family back home flooded me with calls if the news reported any natural disaster within 500 miles. If they heard that 27,000 acres were on fire, it sounded like the entire Golden State rather than a 3-mile radius. In the fall of 2019, when we moved, Ohio was abuzz when our beloved native basketballer LeBron James was forced to evacuate his California estate. I got six calls to assess our safety that day. I found it comical that my friends and family thought I lived anywhere near King James. Uncle Brian didn't share in my amusement and cautioned me that "fires move fast Bridge" with all seriousness while I muffled my snickers with my hand over my mouth and thanked him for his concern.

They say you can't run away from your problems, but maybe you can. Perhaps it's just that you cannot run away from problems you created or patterns you haven't broken. Moving can be a fresh start, a turn toward a new chapter. In some cases, distance can give you clarity and peace. That's what it's done for me, though I recognize it's not feasible for everyone.

I'd lived two hours away from my mother since college, but somehow, I still felt like I couldn't fully escape her shadow. The "grapevine" was too close. The family drama seeped into my world at regular intervals. Debra said this, and Debra did that. Nothing could keep Hurricane Debra at bay.

Then, I moved 2,100 miles away. It was a great career opportunity, but also gave me the psychological freedom to continue evolving outside Mom's shadow. I could better digest her intermittent escapades from afar. With time on my hands due to the pandemic and half a lifetime of material to digest, I was ready to share my story, to lift that invisible weight.

***

Kaliyah was a 31-year-old African American divorced mother of three. She'd been referred to my 4th-year clinical practicum site for court-mandated parenting assessment. During an argument with her 8-year-old daughter, she'd lost control and struck the child over the head with a children's plastic folding chair, knocking her to the floor and leaving a bump on her forehead.

The authorities quickly became involved, and Kaliyah found herself facing severe consequences. She was ordered to participate in an evaluation to determine her mental state and assess her ability to provide a safe and nurturing environment for her children, who were temporarily placed with their father.

Kaliyah was resistant to the evaluation from the start, which is typical for court-mandated clients. The standard rules of doctor–patient confidentiality do not apply, and I was required to submit a detailed report to the court and perhaps testify. The clients see me as a "snitch" before we ever get started. Over 3–4 sessions, I conducted a clinical interview, diagnostic assessment, and personality inventory on Kaliyah.

She had little insight into the severity of the problem, at one point detailing, "My dad used to beat me until I was bloodied and bruised, and no one took him to court." For her, striking a child with the nearest object (e.g., shoe, cup, remote, chair) felt like an acceptable disciplinary practice within her cultural and religious framework, and she demonstrated no remorse.

Kaliyah's test results indicated an average IQ, a history of adverse childhood experiences (ACEs), and hints of a personality disorder. I provided her with a summary of my findings and what disclosures I planned to make to the court. Over the weeks, it had begun to sink in that she could permanently lose custody of her kids. This prospect seemed to frighten her, and she was willing to "do anything" to get them back. Kaliyah appeared amenable to the healthy discipline strategies I provided her, including time-outs, loss of privileges, and behavior contracts.

As we stood from our respective chairs to close our final session, Kaliyah turned to me, eyes burning.

"So, how long are we going to pretend like we don't know each other?"

I narrowed my eyes in confusion.

"You don't ever have to acknowledge me if we see each other in public," I offered, thinking she was referring to future encounters.

"No, I mean the fact that we already know each other."

"We do?" I looked at her face more closely, not finding the faintest glint of familiarity.

"Yes, I came to homecoming once at your church last year with my Aunt Rhonda. I was sitting *right* behind you!"

There were so many odd statements in those two sentences. Once? A year ago? Behind me? Not to mention, 300+ people attended that church on a given Sabbath, let alone a homecoming weekend crowd. She had a different last name than her aunt, whom I did know.

I side-eyed Kaliyah before retaining my therapy poker face.

"I'm sorry, that was so long ago, and I don't remember."

"Oh, okay," she concluded with a sarcastic drip and sashayed toward the door.

Part of me found her accusation humorous, but another piece felt frightened. Why did she remember *me*? My gut burned, telling me I might've missed something. My supervisor and I considered amending my report but we couldn't find the words to account for the odd encounter. We submitted it to the court as written, and it was out of our hands. The court never followed up to share their custody decision. All I could do was send up a prayer for the safety of those children and hope I never ran into her at church again.

***

Among lay audiences, physical abuse is often viewed on a subjective continuum of severity, influenced by arbitrary factors such as personal experiences with corporal punishment, perceptions of intensity, or the victim's age. What we may not realize is how desensitized we have become to recognizing acts of physical abuse or intimidation. A more objective lens is necessary. Instead of relying on personal thresholds, consider these critical questions: Is the act threatening or aggressive? Does it involve physical contact? Did it leave marks, bruises, or have the potential to cause physical harm? These criteria offer a clearer and more consistent framework for identifying physical abuse.

I often witness this in clinical settings with patients grappling with these experiences. They feel the emotional hurt of physical violence but struggle with labeling it as abuse. The case of "Samantha" comes to mind.

Samantha was my doctoral supervisee's patient at a university clinic. With patient consent, I watched the sessions live stream from the next room. Samantha was a 25-year-old, lesbian woman of unknown "mixed" race and the mother of a three-year-old child. She came to therapy to seek support after separating from her wife. Samantha was uncertain about her decision. Fed up with her wife's controlling nature and constant put-downs, Samantha had taken her daughter from a previous relationship and moved in with her mother.

In the session, she easily labeled her wife's name-calling and constant monitoring as emotionally abusive and unacceptable. She then shared that she "went too far" one day. Samantha was in the car with one of her friends when her wife pulled up and began to scream at her through her open window. Samantha drove off, but her estranged wife pursued them. Fearing an accident, she eventually pulled over. Her wife stopped, got out, and approached her car. Samantha thought her wife would continue to argue. Instead, she grabbed Samantha by her hair and pulled her petite frame out the car window and pushed her onto the hood of the car. Samantha finished the story by saying, "I was so embarrassed that my friend saw that."

My supervisee and I were surprised that she had not mentioned physical abuse up to that point. After summarizing her story, my supervisee praised Samantha for being a domestic violence survivor. I watched on the screen as Samantha's demeanor shifted. She sat straight in her chair, cocked her curly head to the side, and looked at my student as if she had two heads.

"No. It wasn't domestic violence. She never punched me in the face."

Samantha indicated this factually and with finality, as if my supervisee had simply misunderstood her story. My supervisee halted in disbelief, unsure as a new trainee where to go next. It was apparent to her (and me, behind the monitor) that this was a case of intimate partner violence (IPV).

Samantha was in denial, a standard tool of psychological self-protection. Denial is an unconscious defense mechanism that causes us to ignore, minimize, or avoid difficult feelings and problems. Her internal ideals of IPV may have been shaped by societal depictions or familial models of abuse, perhaps only in the limited context of heteronormative presentations.[2,3]

My supervisee began the session the following week by checking in regarding how Samantha had been doing since their last meeting. Samantha reported that she'd been toiling over the idea that she had been physically abused, which reopened the door for discussion. With proper therapeutic timing, my student trainee informed Samantha that her response was normal and encouraged her to explore her story in a safe setting to heal. Samantha was open to the treatment plan, including psychoeducation on IPV signs and cycles, safety planning, resource advocacy, and healthy coping strategies to promote healing.

One of the most impactful interventions seemed to be a handout on the varied behaviors that constitute IPV.[4,5] Samantha's eyes widened as she ticked off more than a dozen boxes indicating abusive experiences like pushing, pinching, and restraining from her wife. She went on to journal extensively about these stories and shared them in later sessions. It was something tangible that kept her from rationalizing her experience or counterarguing with stories of her wife's "niceness." In her insightfulness, she'd noticed the progressive pattern of her abuse and saw that it was only getting worse. It strengthened her to name the fire in her gut that told her something was wrong, and she needed to get out. It helped solidify her decision to end the relationship permanently. She made the temporary move to her mother's house permanent. This provided safety, financial backing, and social support, resources some survivors may not have readily accessible. Samantha shared everything that happened with her mother and a trusted girlfriend as a form of external accountability. She also realized the potential impact on her child, who had been sheltered from the abuse up to then. She vowed to protect her.

For the time being, my student trainee and I were relieved, but we also knew that, on average, it takes individuals experiencing IPV seven times before leaving for good.[6] I held my breath, hoping that our early therapeutic interventions and social support from her mother would help Samantha keep her resolve. At least then, she and her child were safe from the flames.

With me, Mom had lit the final match at an early age. I was burning up and realized that no one was going to save me. I could let the fire consume me or harness its power. So, I grabbed the reins of my life. It tested my strength and resilience, but I was tougher than anyone had imagined. They had no idea what I was made of, nor did I. I held on with all my might. The flame never extinguished and only evolved. Ultimately, I became the fire—saving myself and, in turn, my children.

References

1. Smyth, M. R., & Tyson, G. A. (2024). How does denial, minimization, justifying, and blaming operate in intimate partner abuse committed by men: A systematic review of the literature. *Trauma, Violence, & Abuse, 25*(3), 1853–1870. https://doi.org/10.1177/15248380231196108

2. MacDonald, K., Thomas, M. L., Sciolla, A. F., Schneider, B., Pappas, K., Bleijenberg, G., & Wingenfeld, K. (2016). Minimization of childhood maltreatment is common and consequential: Results from a large, multinational sample using the Childhood Trauma Questionnaire. *PLOS ONE, 11*(1), e0146058. https://doi.org/10.1371/journal.pone.0146058

3. DomesticShelters.org. (2023). *"It's really not that bad"—Why some survivors minimize their abuse.* https://www.domesticshelters.org/articles/taking-care-of-you/why-some-survivors-minimize-their-abuse

4. Arizona Coalition to End Sexual and Domestic Violence. (2023). *Types of domestic violence.* https://www.acesdv.org/domestic-violence-graphics/types-of-abuse/

5. Breiding, M. J., Chen, J., & Black, M. C. (2014). *Intimate partner violence in the United States--2010.* https://stacks.cdc.gov/view/cdc/21961

6. World Health Organization (WHO). (2012). *Understanding and addressing violence against women.* https://apps.who.int/iris/bitstream/handle/10665/77432/WHO_RHR_12.36_eng.pdf

CHAPTER 17

Close Encounter

Psychological Closure

Psychological closure involves the integration of traumatic experiences into a coherent narrative, allowing the survivor to reestablish a stable sense of self. Rather than a singular event, closure is often a dynamic process marked by posttraumatic growth, emotional regulation, and the reconstruction of meaning.[1-3]

AFTER GRANNY'S DEATH, it would be six and half years before I'd see Debra again, a forced reunion for Pawpaw's 90th-birthday celebration near the "Most Enjoyable Place on Earth" in hot, humid Orlando, Florida. We'd arrived early to the celebration, bearing bronzed shoulders, care of the California sun, and taking up half a table adjacent to the dance floor. Resisting the stereotype of CPT, colored people time, we'd beaten the guest of honor and were able to celebrate his calm and collected entrance. Soon after Pawpaw's arrival, a long line of late relatives flowed into the room. My heart lifted. I swished across the floor in my strapless, floor-length sun dress and went to greet everyone with hugs and hellos.

I was making my way down the row, excited to see family I hadn't seen in years: my uncle, my cousin, my brother, his wife. I didn't notice her. Maybe it was her back-length strawberry-blond wig that momentarily disguised her. The recent reboot about a defiant mermaid had just been released, and perhaps it was a fitting nod given our location. Or was it her latest way of signaling illness? It was too late when her face and abstract attire finally registered. Debra was next in line.

Part of me wanted to stay true to myself, to turn and walk away. This woman had hardly made it 20 miles to the hospital to visit her dying mother but she'd come 1,000 miles for a party. The other part of me had silently vowed not to inadvertently stir up any family drama on Pawpaw's important day. A hug wouldn't kill me. Debra could no longer hurt me.

"Mom," I stated out of obligation, though she was "Debra" in my heart.

I leaned down, attempting a loose, disconnected, London Bridge-style hug. My arms bent, and I patted the back side of her arms.

Debra stood like a statue. She uttered no words in return. Her arms hung limp at her sides. Her glassy, red eyes looked past me.

A week later, Devon told me she'd had a similar emotionless encounter with Debra that day at the party.

"Aren't I supposed to feel something when I hug my own mother?" Devon pondered.

It had otherwise been a great weekend with normal family discord and fun. Who paid too much, and who didn't. How so-and-so is a better cook than the restaurant chef. How our Uncle Brian doesn't realize that many songs were created after 1996. How I'd scuffed up my new designer sandals on the sticky dance floor. Why our white great aunt thought Devon and I had learned the choreography for standard line dances via video chat for some odd reason. How fun it had been to hang out with our cousins by the pool and talk about our crazy parents. We'd had an amazing but brief time. For me, seeing Debra hadn't registered as a critical event. I tried to reassure my younger sister.

"Maybe not feeling anything is a sign of progress and healing. Mom no longer has an impact on our emotions. There's no optimism or hopefulness or anger and bitterness. Her action or inaction no longer moves us. She is powerless," I offered.

"You're right," Devon agreed. "It is what it is."

We didn't devote an hour to our hurts, recounting stories from our 35 years of abuse like we used to. We didn't wallow in sadness or anger. We didn't place blame. We were gray rocks. We accepted it, a crucial part of closure and recovery. Without this step, unresolved grief can leave survivors trapped in a cycle of conflicting emotions—anger, sadness, guilt, or relief—making closure feel elusive. The pain may fester, leading to ongoing torment or complicated grief should the abuser pass away down the road. By choosing acceptance, you give yourself permission to live outside the shadow of the abuser and to freely build a healthy life of your own.

Mom was now just a person we knew. We shifted to a new topic of discussion, sort of.

"How's the book coming?" Devon asked.

***

In hindsight, something about seeing Debra at that moment felt genuine, authentic, and truthful. It was the most honest response I'd ever gotten from her, like she could finally tell her "truth" too. No more barely veiled disdain, competition, lies, or performative mothering. No forced engagement due to our biological ties. This was who she truly was, cold and distant. It was likely a relief to hate me outright. No more burden of pretend.

It probably felt fair to her to emotionally push me away as I'd done to her out of necessity. In her skewed perspective of the world, I'd wounded her by not succumbing to her will. My boundaries had caused her emotional injury. I'd further denied her access to her grandchildren whom she envisioned she would never harm but whom I knew were not safe in her care. Her retaliatory distance felt somehow just. I was disrespectful and dishonorable ... and I was alright with it. I was healed yet she would forever be the same.

That final encounter affirmed my place of peace. We were finally on the same page. Simply two women, bonded by lineage, unchained by life, and finally letting go of what likely never was, mother and daughter.

References

1. Guha, A. (2021, June 30). How to find psychological closure: Understanding and moving past difficult experiences. *Psychology Today.* https://www.psychologytoday.com/us/blog/prisons-and-pathos/202106/how-find-psychological-closure?msockid=380b5c7fda1165241efe495edb836453

2. Greenberg, L. S. (2015). *Emotion-focused therapy: Coaching clients to work through their feelings.* American Psychological Association.

3. Noonan, S. (2019, December 2). The art of letting go: How letting go of a positive or a negative can impact our lives. https://www.psychologytoday.com/us/blog/view-from-the-mist/201912/the-art-of-letting-go?msockid=380b5c7fda1165241efe495edb836453

"And, ye fathers, provoke not your children to wrath: but bring them up in the nurture and admonition of the Lord."

—Ephesians 6:4 (KJV)

Epilogue

I COLLAPSED ON the bed, exhausted from packing all day. We'd been chugging through the monumental task of upheaving our lives to move across the country. I was grateful that, for this move, the girls were old enough to help organize, box and label their belongings. Through the haze of exhaustion, I noticed someone had left a sizeable stack of torn, 5 × 7 loose-leaf notebook paper on my bed. I didn't inspect it closely as I called them to my bedroom to return their property.

"Did one of you leave these in here?"

The girls looked confused.

"I've never seen those before," Taryn, the oldest, offered with a preteen shrug.

"I thought they were yours," Jordyn replied.

"Why would you think they're mine?"

"I dunno. They're about abuse."

I whipped the pages toward my face, worried that they hid some secret message one of my children was trying to share. The title was direct, a poem called Song of the Abused. It wasn't in either of their handwriting, but I was concerned.

"Where'd you find these?" I asked but was a bit afraid of the answer.

"I pulled out my dresser drawers to pack them, and they fell out."

"Show me."

I walked behind my youngest child to her room, flipping through the mangled pages on our ascent down a flight of stairs. The remaining poems followed the same abusive melody, "A Place that Doesn't Exist," "In Your Darkest Days," and "Invisable." Some were untitled, unfinished. The rushed penmanship and spelling errors made some challenging to discern.

I got down to her room, and the white dresser with purple flowers stood empty. She'd had it since her first "big girl" room as a toddler. It had already survived at least two moves. One from the seller in the online marketplace and another from the townhouse we'd lived in to ensure our children could attend the best schools in the city. The six drawers sat stacked full of clothes in front of the hollow frame.

"They were stuck back there," Jordyn pointed to the top left corner of the unpainted interior.

I crouched down for a closer inspection. Nothing remained except a few scraps of the curly, perforated paper.

The dresser had been a secret hiding spot for someone's untold pain. An unknown girl or young woman had suffered abuse in a similar way as I had. Whether parent or partner, she'd tried to cover her scars and resisted inflicting her own. I felt her pain through those crumpled pages.

I had no way to find her, but I hope she picks up this book and discovers her words here one day. I hope she knows that she is not alone and didn't continue to suffer in silence. I pray she found a way out, got help, and is surviving and thriving. That is my desire for all of us.

With respect for this unnamed writer, I share this piece to honor their voice and the voices of countless others whose pain often goes unseen. It is transcribed as originally written.

Song of the abused
—Author Unknown

the crying screams
the sound of a hit so strong
you know it broke flesh
some hear that sound
and wince in remembrance
bringing back dreadful memories
listening to the child
as they scream
stop, stop, please stop
the sounds of painful sobs
the sound of painful hearts
seeing the child walk out
seeing their tear streaked face
trying to hide their pain
hiding the shaking in their emotion
wanting to hide
but forced to stay in public
the gasping air as people see
the bruises, the scars
bring the sleeves full length
and wear long pants
just to hide that they're beat
the repeated strikes
the often case of bloodshed
leading the victim helpless
often times laying on the floor
limp and lifeless
trying to get away from the attacker
these are the sounds and sites of abuse
this is the song of the abused
this happens every day

Appendix

Adverse Childhood Experiences Screening

Below, you can complete the adverse childhood experiences (ACEs) measure and calculate your score.[1] It is advisable to explore these questions and checklists with the guidance and expertise of a licensed mental health professional. Their support can prove invaluable as clients examine these experiences.

Below is a list of 10 categories of ACEs. Review the list and place a checkmark next to each category that applies to experiences you had before your 18th birthday. Once completed, count the number of categories you marked and record the total at the bottom.
☐   Physical Abuse: Did a parent or other adult in the household often or very often ... Push, grab, slap, or throw something at you? Or Ever hit you so hard that you had marks or were injured?
☐   Emotional or Psychological Abuse: Did a parent or other adult in the household often or very often ... Swear at you, insult you, put you down, or humiliate you? Or Act in a way that made you afraid that you might be physically hurt?
☐   Sexual Abuse: Did an adult or person at least five years older than you ever ... Touch or fondle you or have you touch their body in a sexual way? Or attempt or actually have oral, anal, or vaginal intercourse with you?
☐   Physical Neglect: Did you often or very often feel that ... You didn't have enough to eat, had to wear dirty clothes, and had no one to protect you? Or your parents were too drunk or high to take care of you or take you to the doctor if you needed it?
☐   Emotional Neglect: Did you feel that no one in your family loved you or thought you were special? Or your family didn't look out for each other, feel close to each other, or support each other?

(dis)Honor Thy Mother: Daughterhood, Dysfunction and Deliverance, First Edition. Bridgette Peteet.
© 2026 John Wiley & Sons, Inc. Published 2026 by John Wiley & Sons, Inc.

☐ Household Mental Illness: Was a household member depressed or mentally ill, or did a household member attempt suicide?
☐ Domestic Violence: Was your mother or stepmother: Often or very often pushed, grabbed, slapped, or had something thrown at her? Or sometimes, often, or very often kicked, bitten, hit with a fist, or hit with something hard? Or ever repeatedly hit over at least a few minutes or threatened with a gun or knife?
☐ Parental Separation or Divorce or Death: Were your parents ever separated or divorced?
☐ Household Member Incarceration: Did a household member go to prison?
☐ Household Substance Abuse: Did you live with anyone who was a problem drinker or alcoholic, or who used street drugs?
____ Your ACE score is the total number of categories you checked.

Interpreting Your ACEs Score

Remember that not all ACEs carry the same weight. This scale also does not measure the frequency or severity of events. Here's a breakdown of the scores:

- *0 ACEs:* Indicates no reported experiences of the listed adverse events. This suggests a lower likelihood of long-term negative health and behavioral outcomes but does not eliminate the possibility of other challenges.
- *1–3 ACEs:* Represents some exposure to adversity. Individuals in this range may experience mild to moderate impacts, depending on protective factors like supportive relationships or coping mechanisms.
- *4 or More ACEs:* Indicates significant exposure to adversity, which research links to a higher risk of physical and mental health issues, including chronic disease, depression, anxiety, and substance use disorders (SUDs).

It's important to note that while a higher ACE score correlates with increased risk, it is not deterministic. Protective factors, such as strong support systems, access to resources, and resilience-building practices, can mitigate the negative effects of ACEs.

Source of ACEs

Who was the primary person(s) responsible for the experiences of ACEs identified in the previous section? (Select all that apply):

- ☐ Father
- ☐ Mother
- ☐ Stepfather
- ☐ Stepmother
- ☐ Other family member (e.g., grandparent, uncle/aunt, cousin)
- ☐ Caregiver/foster parent/adoptive parent
- ☐ Other: _____

Understanding the source of child abuse is crucial in addressing its impact and creating effective intervention strategies.[2] Society often associates abuse more prominently with fathers or male figures, aligning with stereotypes of men as authoritarian or physically aggressive.[3] This narrative, while not untrue, can overshadow the abuse perpetrated by mothers, which is less frequently discussed due to societal expectations of mothers as nurturing caregivers.[4] Maternal abuse, including emotional neglect, verbal abuse, or physical harm, can be particularly damaging because it contradicts societal ideals, leaving survivors with a complex mix of shame, confusion, and self-doubt.[5]

Similarly, abuse by stepparents may be underreported or minimized, as blended families face unique challenges that can obscure harmful dynamics.[6] Children in these situations might feel pressure to accept the new family structure or fear that speaking out could disrupt relationships further.[7] Recognizing these patterns is critical for breaking stigmas and ensuring all forms of abuse are acknowledged. By addressing the nuances of abuse sources—including gender roles, societal expectations, and family dynamics—advocates, clinicians, and communities can better support survivors and create more inclusive approaches to prevention and intervention.[8]

References

1. Centers for Disease Control and Prevention (CDC). (n.d.). *Fast facts: Preventing adverse childhood experiences.* https://www.cdc.gov/violenceprevention/aces/fastfact.html
2. Cicchetti, D., & Toth, S. L. (2005). Child maltreatment. *Annual Review of Clinical Psychology, 1*(1), 409–438. https://doi.org/10.1146/annurev.clinpsy.1.102803.144029
3. Scantlebury, A., Negriff, S., & Trickett, P. K. (2021). Gender differences in child maltreatment experiences: Implications for developmental trajectories. *Child Abuse & Neglect, 119,* 104733. https://doi.org/10.1016/j.chiabu.2021.104733
4. Chan, K. L., Brownridge, D. A., Yan, E., & Ip, P. (2022). Maternal versus paternal perpetration of child maltreatment: Examining risks and consequences. *Journal of Interpersonal Violence, 37*(1–2), NP104–NP126. https://doi.org/10.1177/0886260519898443
5. Freyd, J. J. (1996). *Betrayal trauma: The logic of forgetting childhood abuse.* Harvard University Press.
6. Sweeney, S., Toth, S. L., & Cicchetti, D. (2019). The impact of stepfamily dynamics on child maltreatment: Risks and resilience. *Development and Psychopathology, 31*(2), 601–616. https://doi.org/10.1017/S0954579418001002
7. Platt, V. B., Freyd, J. J., & Birrell, P. J. (2018). Betrayal trauma and institutional betrayal in foster care settings: When caregiving fails. *Psychological Trauma Theory Research Practice and Policy, 10*(1), 102–109. https://doi.org/10.1037/tra0000257
8. Font, S. A., & Maguire-Jack, K. (2020). The scope, nature, and causes of child abuse and neglect. *The Annals of the American Academy of Political and Social Science, 692*(1), 26–49. https://doi.org/10.1177/0002716220969642

ACEs Prevalence, Examples, and Intervention Strategies

Based on your responses to the items above, the following section offers deeper insights into the prevalence of each type of abuse, along with examples that you may or may not have considered. Each section concludes with practical strategies designed to help readers provide support and foster healing for children who have experienced abuse.

ACE: Physical Abuse

Child physical abuse is when a parent or adult caregiver inflicts intentional or malicious injury. It also includes failure to protect a child from physical abuse.[1] Global estimates suggest that 22% of children experience physical abuse.[2] Physical abuse differs from corporal punishment, which is any use of force to correct behavior, however mild.[3] Global UNICEF data show that approximately 60% of children experienced corporal punishment in the past month.[4] Even making this distinction is problematic because studies indicate that spanking increases the odds of physical abuse.[5,6]

Though the boundaries between physical abuse and punishment may be blurry, the main distinguishing factors are severity, intention, and intervention. This includes bodily location, use of objects, excessiveness, frequency, repetitiveness, intensity, and maliciousness.[7] Law enforcement and child protective services are more likely to intervene in physical abuse cases than corporal punishment.[1]

Studies show that neither physical abuse nor corporal punishment yields long-term positive outcomes and is no more effective than other forms of discipline.[3,8] Using force leads to lasting negative effects such as increased risk-taking behaviors, aggression, delinquency, and substance abuse.[9]

Examples of Physical Abuse:

❑ Abuse of pets	❑ Hitting with objects	❑ Shaking
❑ Being thrown	❑ Kicking	❑ Shooting
❑ Biting	❑ Red marks infliction	❑ Shoving
❑ Broken bones	❑ Welts infliction	❑ Slapping
❑ Bruising	❑ Locked out of the house or in the house	❑ Sleep deprivation
❑ Burning	❑ Nipping	❑ Snatching
❑ Choking or strangling	❑ Physical restraint	❑ Spanking with hand or small object
❑ Cutting	❑ Poisoning	❑ Spitting
❑ Destroying property	❑ Pulling hair	❑ Squeezing
❑ Driving dangerously	❑ Punching	❑ Stabbing
❑ Food deprivation	❑ Pushing	❑ Suffocating
❑ Forced feeding	❑ Restraining	❑ Throwing things
❑ Grabbing	❑ Scalding	
❑ Head butting	❑ Scratching	
❑ Hitting with hands		

Alternatives to corporal punishment focus on nurturing discipline strategies that promote emotional intelligence, respect, and accountability. These include setting clear expectations, using time-outs effectively, implementing logical and natural consequences, and fostering open communication. For example, a parent can encourage a child to reflect on their actions by asking questions like, "What could you do differently next time?" or "How can we fix this together?" Positive reinforcement, such as praising desired behaviors, also helps build a child's self-esteem and motivates them to make better choices. By choosing these approaches, parents can guide their children with love and consistency, ensuring discipline becomes an opportunity for growth rather than fear.

ACE: Emotional Abuse

Childhood emotional abuse, also called psychological abuse, is a recurring trauma in which the parent verbally abuses, ignores, humiliates, or intimidates to control a child. Some estimates suggest that 2–10% of children have experienced emotional abuse, but these numbers may be low since this form of abuse is more difficult to detect.[10,11] As an ACE, emotional abuse includes a range of verbal and nonverbal messages that the child is unloved or worthless. It damages a child's sense of well-being and self-worth and can cause deep emotional wounds.[12] Emotional abuse is often accompanied by more obvious abuse, including physical abuse, sexual abuse, and child neglect.[13]

Emotional abuse is also unlike other forms of abuse in many ways. Some argue that it is more psychologically harmful than physical abuse.[14,15] Since the acts are less obvious, they are less noticeable and more likely to go unreported. Survivors of emotional abuse are also more likely to turn pain inward and blame themselves than with physical abuse, where they may see more clearly that the fault is external.[16] Emotional abuse is also more likely to continue when the child becomes an adult, manifesting in emotionally abusive relationships or parenting behaviors.[17]

There are numerous signs of emotional abuse, such as low self-esteem, anxiety, withdrawal, and increased fear. Emotionally abused children may seem too competent and mature or too young and childlike for their age. As adults, they may engage in unhealthy coping strategies such as substance abuse and have mental health problems.[18] Survivors may unintentionally end up in emotionally abusive relationships as adults or emotionally abusing their children.[19]

Examples of Emotional Abuse:

❏ Accusing	❏ Indifference	❏ Shame
❏ Blaming	❏ Insults (physical, intellectual)	❏ Shutting down communication
❏ Control	❏ Isolation	
❏ Dehumanizing	❏ Jealousy	❏ Swearing at you
❏ Denying	❏ Lecturing	❏ Threats
❏ Denying abuse occurred	❏ Name-calling (needy, no sense of humor)	❏ Turning the tables (you are the cause)
❏ Dismissiveness		
❏ Disputing your feelings	❏ Pushing your buttons	❏ Unpredictability
❏ Fist pounding	❏ Put-downs of your interests	❏ Withholding affection
❏ Gaslighting	❏ Sarcasm	
❏ Humiliation	❏ Screaming	

Breaking the cycle of emotional abuse involves adopting nurturing, affirming, and constructive communication strategies that foster a child's emotional well-being. Instead of criticism or ridicule, parents can practice positive reinforcement by acknowledging and celebrating their child's efforts and achievements, no matter how small. When a child makes a mistake, reframing the situation as a learning opportunity encourages growth rather than shame. Open-ended questions like, "How are you feeling about this?" or "What can we do to solve this together?" invite dialogue and build problem-solving skills. Setting boundaries with empathy—explaining the "why" behind rules and consequences—creates a sense of fairness and respect. Additionally, modeling emotional regulation, such as calmly expressing frustrations without yelling or resorting to blame, teaches children how to navigate their own emotions healthily. Through patience, compassion, and intentional connection, parents can create a nurturing environment that supports healing and builds trust.

ACE: Sexual Abuse

Child sexual abuse is the involvement of a child in sexual activity that they may not fully comprehend, are unable to give informed consent to, or for which they are not developmentally prepared and cannot give consent, or that violates the laws or social taboos of society.[19] These acts can be physical (e.g., sexual touching, intercourse) or emotional (e.g., exposure to pornography) and occur within same-sex or mixed-gender interactions. There are degrees of severity (e.g., violent, stranger, long-term), but all sexual abuse is wrong, harmful, and confusing for children.

Sexual abuse is not an easy subject to discuss. It is a painful and traumatic experience that affects many families. About one in five (21%) of children are sexual abuse victims. One in 5 girls and 1 in 20 boys experience this type of abuse.[20–22] Most abused children are familiar with their perpetrators and are likelier to be family, friends of the family, neighbors, or other trusted adults rather than strangers.[23]

Behavioral change can often be a significant and concerning sign of child sexual abuse. Children are typically resilient and adaptable, but when they undergo such traumatic experiences, they may exhibit a range of noticeable behavioral alterations. These shifts can manifest in various ways, from becoming withdrawn or unusually secretive to displaying excessive aggression or fear. Moreover, changes in self-esteem, sudden aversion to specific people or places, or the emergence of age-inappropriate sexual knowledge or behaviors can all be alarming indicators.[24,25] These transformations are often an outward reflection of the internal turmoil and distress caused by the abuse, and they underscore the critical importance of carefully monitoring and supporting children who might be experiencing abuse.

Examples of Childhood Sexual Abuse:

☐ *Touching:* Inappropriate touching of a child's private parts or forcing a child to touch an adult's private parts.
☐ *Fondling:* Repeatedly fondling a child's genitals, breasts, or buttocks for sexual gratification.
☐ *Oral–Genital Contact:* Forcing a child to perform or receive oral sex.
☐ *Penetration:* Any form of vaginal, anal, or oral penetration of a child by an adult or an older child.
☐ *Exhibitionism:* Exposing a child to sexual acts or pornography.
☐ *Child Pornography:* Creating, sharing, or possessing explicit images or videos of minors.
☐ *Online Exploitation:* Grooming a child for sexual purposes through online communication or coercion.
☐ *Child Prostitution or Sex Trafficking:* Forcing or coercing a child into commercial sex acts.

Preventing child sexual abuse begins with creating a foundation of trust, education, and open communication from parents.[26–28] Parents and caregivers can empower children by teaching them about body autonomy and the concept of consent from an early age. This includes using proper names for body parts, which removes shame and confusion, and reinforcing that their body belongs to them. Encourage children to speak up if they feel uncomfortable, emphasizing that secrets about touch are never okay, and that they will always be believed and supported. Parents should also establish clear boundaries with other adults and model respectful behavior in their own interactions. Regularly monitoring and staying engaged in a child's activities—both in person and online—helps identify potential risks. It is equally important to educate oneself about the signs of grooming and abuse while fostering an environment where a child feels safe to discuss any concerns. By prioritizing education, vigilance, and trust, families can significantly reduce the risk of abuse and equip children with tools to protect themselves.

ACE: Physical Neglect

Physical neglect is the deprivation of basic needs such as food, clothing, and shelter. It also includes educational, environmental, medical, and supervisory neglect.[29] Educational neglect is the failure to provide appropriate access to education, while environmental neglect occurs when a child's surroundings threaten their health and safety. Medical neglect involves failing to address a child's medical needs or disregarding medical advice. Supervisory neglect refers to the failure to adequately monitor or protect a child from harm.[30]

These types of neglect are not always tied to financial hardship. For instance, some abusive parents may deliberately withhold basic necessities as a form of punishment or to conceal abuse.[31] In other cases, however, poverty contributes significantly to physical neglect. Families living in food deserts may lack access to affordable, nutritious food, a situation stemming not from choice but from systemic inequities in access and infrastructure.[32]

Despite the overall wealth of the United States, child poverty remains alarmingly high. More than 11 million children (16%) live in poverty.[33] Women and racial/ethnic minorities are disproportionately represented among those experiencing poverty due to structural racism and gender inequality.[34,35] Research has established a strong correlation between childhood adversity and poverty; in fact, some experts argue that poverty itself constitutes a distinct ACE, beyond the other recognized forms of neglect.[36,37] Although poverty is associated with increased risk for ACEs, it is not a direct cause and many low-income families provide nurturing, stable environments for their children.[38]

Examples of Physical Neglect:

- ☐ Insufficient shelter
- ☐ Frequent housing changes
- ☐ Filthy home environment
- ☐ Animal infestations
- ☐ Inadequate food
- ☐ Rotten food
- ☐ Non-nutritious food
- ☐ Inadequate clean water
- ☐ Inaccessible nonfood goods
- ☐ Insufficient clothing
- ☐ Unclean clothing
- ☐ Inhibited access to healthcare
- ☐ Irregular school attendance
- ☐ Failure to register
- ☐ Chronic absenteeism/truancy
- ☐ Low parental monitoring

Addressing child physical neglect starts with ensuring families have access to resources that meet their basic needs, such as food, housing, healthcare, and education. Often rooted in systemic inequities like poverty, unemployment, or lack of access to social services, solutions require both immediate interventions and long-term support.[31] Community programs, food banks, and housing assistance initiatives can provide critical relief to families in crisis, while advocacy for policies that improve wages, childcare access, and affordable healthcare can address root causes.[32,34]

Parents and caregivers may also benefit from parenting education programs that teach budgeting, nutrition, and home safety, as well as counseling to address underlying stressors or trauma that contribute to neglect.[30] Building a support network of trusted friends, family, and community members helps reduce caregiver isolation and provides additional oversight and care for children.

ACE: Emotional Neglect

Emotional neglect occurs when a child's emotional needs for love, support, and attention are consistently unmet by caregivers.[39] It is more common than many realize, with studies suggesting that approximately 18% of children may experience some form of emotional neglect.[40] The impact on children can be profound and long lasting, affecting their ability to form healthy relationships, regulate emotions, and develop a strong sense of self-worth.[41] Emotionally neglected children may struggle with anxiety, depression, and a heightened risk of substance use or other maladaptive coping mechanisms in adulthood.[15] They often internalize the neglect, believing they are unworthy of care or attention, which perpetuates cycles of low self-esteem.[42] Unlike physical neglect, emotional neglect is often invisible and can be harder to identify.[40]

Examples of Emotional Neglect:

- ☐ *Ignoring Emotional Needs:* Failing to notice or respond when a child is sad, scared, or in need of comfort.
- ☐ *Withholding Affection:* Rarely expressing love, hugging, or showing warmth toward the child.
- ☐ *Minimizing Feelings:* Dismissing a child's emotions with phrases like "You're overreacting" or "Stop being so sensitive."
- ☐ *Lack of Encouragement:* Neglecting to celebrate a child's achievements or encourage their goals and interests.
- ☐ *Absence of Praise:* Failing to acknowledge or validate a child's efforts or accomplishments, leading them to feel unseen or unimportant.
- ☐ *Emotional Unavailability:* Being physically present but emotionally distant or disengaged, such as through excessive phone use or prioritizing work over interactions with the child.
- ☐ *Inconsistent Emotional Responses:* Being warm and supportive at times but cold and indifferent at others, leaving the child unsure of how to seek support.
- ☐ *Failure to Provide Guidance:* Not teaching the child how to identify, express, or manage their emotions in healthy ways.
- ☐ *Ignoring or Punishing Vulnerability:* Shaming or scolding a child for crying, expressing fear, or asking for help.
- ☐ *No Safe Space for Sharing:* Creating an environment where the child feels they must suppress their emotions to avoid conflict, criticism, or neglect.

Combating childhood emotional neglect begins with fostering an environment of emotional availability, validation, and connection.[43] Caregivers can prioritize attuning to a child's emotional needs by actively listening, showing empathy, and responding with warmth and understanding. Simple acts like acknowledging a child's feelings—saying, "I see you're upset, let's talk about it"—can make a profound difference. Establishing consistent routines for quality time, such as shared meals or bedtime conversations, helps build a sense of safety and trust. Teaching emotional literacy is equally important; caregivers can model how to identify and express feelings, encouraging children to do the same. Seeking support through parenting programs, therapy, or community resources can equip caregivers with tools to break patterns of neglect, especially if they experienced emotional neglect themselves.[44] Ultimately, combating emotional neglect requires intentionality and care, ensuring children grow up feeling seen, valued, and supported in their emotional and developmental journey.

ACE: Mental Illness

Mental illness involves a variety of mood, cognitive, and behavioral limitations that usually impair social, family, or work functioning. There are more than 150 disorders recognized in the field of mental health.[45] Approximately 23% of adults living in the United States reported having a mental disorder in the past year.[46] Without training, it might be hard to answer whether or not a parental figure had a mental illness.

Psychologists most commonly treat anxiety and depression, followed by trauma, personality disorders, and substance abuse.[47] Unfortunately, mental health and treatment are often stigmatized, particularly in minoritized communities.[48] Stigma impacts our ability to recognize when symptoms are severe, last too long, or destroy lives.

Below are some guidelines to help determine when to see a therapist. I believe therapy should be like going to the dentist or the eye doctor, a part of a routine check of our health and well-being. However, I recognize that there are also economic, access, and other barriers to help-seeking. Identification is a helpful first step in improving mental health. Here are some things to look out for:

Signs of Mental Illness:

* *Disclaimer:* This list is not intended to be diagnostic. Please seek the assistance of a qualified mental health professional for further guidance.

- ☐ Significant psychological impairment (e.g., hallucinations, suicidal thoughts)
- ☐ Trouble managing stress, emotions, mood, or thinking
- ☐ Repeated impaired relationships or job performance
- ☐ Inability to cope with significant life transitions (e.g., death, illness)
- ☐ Trauma experience (past or present)
- ☐ Significant changes in sleep, appetite, or interest in activities
- ☐ Use of unhealthy coping skills (e.g., substance misuse, self-harm)

Children coping with parental mental illness often experience confusion, fear, or misplaced guilt, making it crucial to provide them with understanding, support, and tools to navigate their emotions.[49] Open communication is key. Using age-appropriate language, explain that their parent's behavior or mood is due to an illness, not something the child has caused. Encourage children to express their feelings through conversation, art, or journaling, and validate their emotions without judgment. Providing structure and consistency in daily routines can create a sense of stability amid unpredictability.

Connecting children with supportive adults, such as relatives, teachers, or mentors, offers them additional sources of comfort and guidance. Therapy or support groups specifically for children in similar situations can help them feel less isolated and provide strategies to build resilience. Teaching them self-care skills, like relaxation techniques or healthy coping mechanisms, ensures they have tools to manage stress. By fostering an environment of openness, safety, and external support, children can develop the resilience needed to thrive despite the challenges of parental mental illness.

ACE: Abused Parent/Domestic Violence

Violence in the household involves witnessing or being directly exposed to physical or emotional abuse between adults, typically between parents and caregivers. In the United States, approximately 10 million women and men experience intimate partner violence (IPV) annually.[50] Women report more IPV than do men; over 35% of women and 28% of men have experienced rape, physical violence, and/or stalking by an intimate partner in their lifetime.[51] Black and Latina women are more likely to report IPV than do White women.[50] Many IPV survivors also have children who are at risk for abuse.

Witnessing domestic violence affects children in many ways. Studies indicate that in households with IPV, there is a significant likelihood of co-occurring child abuse.[52] Even when not directly targeted, children may experience emotionally distant and unresponsive parenting. These children may become fearful, guilty, anxious, and depressed, or act out in temperamental or antisocial ways. Boys may become abusive men or victims themselves, and girls are more likely to be victims in adulthood, perpetuating the cycle.[53]

It is common to focus only on the extreme behaviors of domestic violence and consequently miss the preceding acts. Physical domestic violence occurs on a continuum. Emotional abuse and isolation typically precede physical assaults. Early assaults may include pushing, slapping, and throwing objects. Later, the acts might progress to punching, kicking, and choking. At the end of the spectrum, it can include assault with weapons and even death. At each progressive stage, the pattern reinforces the abuse.

While it might seem straightforward for most individuals to end a relationship after the first instance of physical violence, the reality of physical abuse often involves a gradual and unpredictable pattern. This pattern can psychologically condition victims to accept violent behavior over time, increasing the likelihood that they will stay in the relationship. The intervals between abusive incidents can vary widely, spanning from weeks to years. This variability may lead survivors to believe the abuse has stopped. On average, it takes survivors approximately 7–12 attempts before they are able to leave permanently—if they are able to at all.[54]

Cycle of Domestic Violence

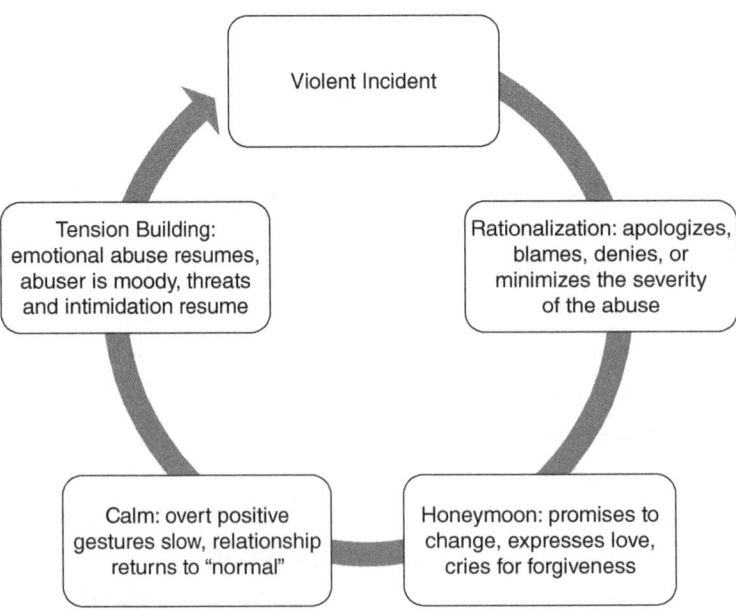

Creating safe spaces for children exposed to domestic violence is essential for their emotional and physical well-being. A safe space begins with a consistent, violence-free environment where children can feel secure and are protected from harm. This might mean removing the child from the abusive household, if possible, or designating a specific area within the home, such as their bedroom, where they can retreat during conflicts, equipped with comforting items like toys, blankets, or books. Open, judgment-free communication is another key component; let the child know it's safe to share their feelings and that their experiences will be met with love, not blame.

Trusted adults, such as relatives, teachers, or counselors, can provide additional safe spaces where the child feels heard and valued. Outside the home, involving children in extracurricular activities or support groups creates opportunities for connection and stability in environments free from violence. Ultimately, ensuring the child knows they are not responsible for the conflict and that they are surrounded by people committed to their safety and well-being lays the foundation for healing and resilience.[53]

ACE: Parental Separation or Divorce

Recent data suggests that the U.S. divorce rate for first-time marriages hit a new low at 39%, rather than the mythical 50% we used to hear.[55] However, the odds of divorce grow to 67% and 74% for second and third marriages, respectively.[56]

Divorce can be confusing and difficult for children, but there are mixed reviews on how it affects them. Children of divorce are more likely to get divorced themselves.[57] However, this remains true of high-conflict households with parents who stay together. Children of multiple divorces tend to be less well adjusted.[58] They may have trouble choosing partners later in life and have difficulty sustaining relationships.[58]

According to research, a "non-parental figure" living in the home is often cited as one of the strongest predictors of child abuse, particularly when compared to a household with only biological parents present.[59] The presence of a nonparental caregiver, especially male, can increase the risk of maltreatment due to potential instability in caregiving dynamics and less established parental bonds.[59]

A nonparental figure may not have the same level of emotional connection and commitment to a child as a biological parent, potentially leading to less attentive care and increased risk of abuse. The presence of a nonparental caregiver can sometimes introduce additional stress within the household, which can contribute to abusive behaviors. Depending on the situation, a nonparental figure might not have the same level of supervision abilities as a biological parent, potentially leading to situations where abuse could occur. While a nonparental figure can be a significant risk factor, it's crucial to remember that not all nonparental caregivers will abuse children.

Learning to choose healthy partners is not always easy, especially if you have had very few models. However, here are some things to consider:

- ☐ Avoid rushing to commitment; people who date three years or longer are 39% less likely to divorce.
- ☐ Do you have lingering strong positive or negative feelings toward your ex or past relationships?
- ☐ Are there excessive personality or behavioral deficits of partner (e.g., immaturity, lying, jealousy, substance abuse, put-downs, isolation from family)?
- ☐ Do you have dissimilar values, goals, and interests?
- ☐ Does your partner have poor conflict resolution skills (e.g., unwilling to compromise, conflict avoidance)?
- ☐ Is there a strained or absent relationship with the current or future family?
- ☐ Few or no external friendships may indicate poor social skills or potential for clinginess
- ☐ Ongoing financial instability (e.g., overspending, debt) is a red flag.
- ☐ Do family/friends voice objections to the union?
- ☐ Is there low commitment to the relationship? Active relationship engagement is necessary for success.

ACE: Incarcerated Family Member

The United States has the world's highest incarceration rate, with over 2 million people currently imprisoned.[60] A significant portion of those incarcerated are parents. In fact, the majority of individuals who are incarcerated have underage children, and one in 25 children is separated from a parent due to incarceration.[61] This statistic highlights a growing but often overlooked issue: the hidden consequences of mass incarceration on children and families. While the criminal justice system focuses on the individual offenders, the impact on their families, particularly their children, is profound and far reaching.[62]

Children of incarcerated parents face a range of emotional, psychological, and social challenges that can have lasting effects on their development. Studies have shown that these children experience higher rates of health and behavioral issues, including anxiety, depression, and trauma-related disorders.[63] The absence of a parent due to incarceration often leads to feelings of abandonment, stigma, and confusion, which can manifest in difficulties with attachment and trust. Furthermore, these children tend to have lower educational attainment, as they may struggle with concentration, performance, and engagement at school due to the stress and instability at home.[64] This can perpetuate a cycle of economic disadvantage, as these children are more likely to experience poverty and fewer opportunities for upward mobility.[62]

In addition to the emotional and psychological strain, children of incarcerated parents often lack the necessary social and economic support systems to offset these negative outcomes. The loss of a parent can lead to financial instability, which in turn affects the child's access to quality education, healthcare, and extracurricular activities that foster positive development. To mitigate these challenges, children in these situations require strong social support networks, including extended family, community resources, and schools that are equipped to offer additional emotional and academic assistance. In many cases, schools and communities must step in to provide these children with the stability and encouragement that may be lacking at home. Addressing the hidden consequences of incarceration requires a more holistic approach to criminal justice reform—one that considers not only the incarcerated individuals but also the children and families who bear the brunt of the consequences.[62]

ACE: Substance Use Disorders

Approximately 20% of children in the United States live in households where at least one parent struggles with alcohol or drug misuse.[65] These environments can be emotionally and psychologically destabilizing. While traditional forms of substance misuse, such as alcohol or illicit drug use, are often more visible, prescription drug misuse may go undetected for longer periods, despite having similarly impairing effects.[66] Substance use can impair a parent's ability to provide consistent, nurturing care, often resulting in emotional unavailability, neglect, or erratic behavior.[67] This disruption to the child's stability and safety can impair their development and contribute to long-term psychological consequences.

Children of parents with SUDs are at elevated risk for emotional and behavioral difficulties, including anxiety, depression, and low self-esteem. Academic struggles, including poor concentration, performance issues, and behavioral disruptions in school, are also common.[68] These children may internalize their distress, withdrawing or acting out, and are more likely to adopt maladaptive coping strategies—including substance use—as they grow older.[69] The intergenerational cycle of addiction and emotional turmoil underscores the urgency of early support and intervention.[70]

Common Signs and Symptoms of Drug Misuse
Risk-Taking Behaviors:

☐ Engaging in dangerous activities such as driving under the influence or having unprotected sex while using substances.

Neglect of Responsibilities:

☐ Failing to meet obligations at school, work, or home due to substance use.

Legal Troubles:

☐ Encounters with law enforcement, such as arrests for disorderly conduct, driving under the influence, or other drug-related offenses.

Physical Warning Signs of Drug Abuse:

☐ Bloodshot eyes or pupils that are unusually large or small.
☐ Noticeable changes in appetite, sleep patterns, or physical appearance.
☐ Unusual smells on the breath, body, or clothing, or impaired coordination.

Behavioral Signs of Drug Abuse:

☐ A decline in attendance or performance at school, work, or social events.
☐ Engaging in secretive, suspicious, or evasive behaviors.
☐ Abrupt changes in friends, hangout spots, or interests.

Psychological Warning Signs of Drug Abuse:

☐ Unexplained shifts in personality or attitude.
☐ Sudden mood swings, irritability, or episodes of being spaced out, angry, or overly defensive.
☐ Exhibiting signs of fear, anxiety, or paranoia without an apparent cause.

Supporting children of parents with SUDs involves creating structured and nurturing environments that foster emotional safety. Establishing consistent routines, such as regular meals and bedtimes, can offer stability.[65] Encouraging open communication, validating emotions, and teaching healthy coping mechanisms (e.g., deep breathing, journaling) help children process their experiences.[67] Trusted adults, including relatives, mentors, and school counselors, can offer added layers of support. Therapy and support groups designed for children of substance-involved parents can reduce isolation and provide tools for resilience.[70] Where substance use creates safety risks, it is vital to establish clear protective plans. By reinforcing the message that addiction is a disease and not the child's fault, caregivers and communities can help these children heal.[71]

References

1. U.S. Department of Health & Human Services, Administration for Children and Families, Children's Bureau. (2023). *Child maltreatment 2021.* https://www.acf.hhs.gov/cb/data-research/child-maltreatment

2. Hillis, S., Mercy, J., Amobi, A., & Kress, H. (2016). Global prevalence of past-year violence against children: A systematic review and minimum estimates. *Pediatrics, 137*(3), e20154079. https://doi.org/10.1542/peds.2015-4079

3. Gershoff, E. T., & Grogan-Kaylor, A. (2016). Spanking and child outcomes: Old controversies and new meta-analyses. *Journal of Family Psychology, 30*(4), 453–469. https://doi.org/10.1037/fam0000191

4. UNICEF (2017). *A familiar face: Violence in the lives of children and adolescents.* United Nations Children's Fund. https://www.unicef.org/publications/index_101397.html

5. Gershoff, E. T. (2013). Spanking and child development: We know enough now to stop hitting our children. *Child Development Perspectives, 7*(3), 133–137. https://doi.org/10.1111/cdep.12038

6. Ma, J., Grogan-Kaylor, A. C., Pace, G. T., Ward, K. P., & Lee, S. J. (2022). The association between spanking and physical abuse of young children in 56 low-and middle-income countries. *Child Abuse & Neglect, 129*, 105662.

7. Font, S. A., & Gershoff, E. T. (2020). Corporal punishment and children's development. *Pediatrics, 145*(6), e20193165. https://doi.org/10.1542/peds.2019-3165

8. Durrant, J., & Ensom, R. (2012). Physical punishment of children: Lessons from 20 years of research. *CMAJ, 184*(12), 1373–1377.

9. Afifi, T. O., Ford, D., Gershoff, E. T., Merrick, M., Grogan-Kaylor, A., Ports, K. A., ... Peters Bennett, R. (2017). Spanking and adult mental health impairment: The case for the designation of spanking as an adverse childhood experience. *Child Abuse & Neglect, 71*, 24–31. https://doi.org/10.1016/j.chiabu.2017.01.014

10. Callaghan, J. E. M., Alexander, J. H., Sixsmith, J., & Fellin, L. C. (2015). Beyond "witnessing": Children's experiences of coercive control in domestic violence and abuse. *Journal of Interpersonal Violence, 33*(10), 1551–1581. https://doi.org/10.1177/0886260515618946

11. Infurna, M. R., Reichl, C., Parzer, P., Schimmenti, A., Bifulco, A., & Brunner, R. (2016). Associations between depression and specific childhood experiences of abuse and neglect: A meta-analysis. *Journal of Affective Disorders, 190*, 47–55. https://doi.org/10.1016/j.jad.2015.09.006

12. Litrownik, A. J., Newton, R. R., Hunter, W. M., English, D., & Everson, M. D. (2015). Exposure to family violence in young at-risk children: A longitudinal look at the effects of victimization and witnessed physical and psychological aggression. *Journal of Interpersonal Violence, 30*(1), 60–79. https://doi.org/10.1177/0886260514535267

13. Lorenc, T., Lester, S., Sutcliffe, K., Stansfield, C., Thomas, J., & Harden, A. (2020). Interventions to support people exposed to adverse childhood experiences: Systematic review of systematic reviews. *BMC Public Health, 20*, 657. https://doi.org/10.1186/s12889-020-08789-0

14. Martins, C. M., Fernandes, M., Soares, I., Veríssimo, M., & Silva, J. R. (2021). Long-term consequences of emotional abuse in childhood: A longitudinal study of adult attachment and well-being. *Child Abuse & Neglect, 114*, 104997. https://doi.org/10.1016/j.chiabu.2021.104997

15. Norman, R. E., Byambaa, M., De, R., Butchart, A., Scott, J., & Vos, T. (2016). The long-term health consequences of child physical abuse, emotional abuse, and neglect: A systematic review and meta-analysis. *PLoS Medicine, 9*(11), e1001349. https://doi.org/10.1371/journal.pmed.1001349

16. Spinazzola, J., Hodgdon, H., Liang, L. J., Ford, J. D., Layne, C. M., Pynoos, R., ... van der Kolk, B. A. (2014). Unseen wounds: The contribution of psychological maltreatment to child and adolescent mental health and risk outcomes. *Psychological Trauma Theory Research Practice and Policy, 6*(Suppl 1), S18–S28. https://doi.org/10.1037/a0037766

17. Teicher, M. H., & Samson, J. A. (2016). Annual research review: Enduring neurobiological effects of childhood abuse and neglect. *Journal of Child Psychology and Psychiatry, 57*(3), 241–266. https://doi.org/10.1111/jcpp.12507

18. van Harmelen, A. L., Gibson, J. L., St Clair, M. C., Owens, M., Brodbeck, J., Dunn, V., ... Goodyer, I. M. (2016). Friendships and family support reduce subsequent depressive symptoms in at-risk adolescents. *PLoS One, 11*(5), e0153715. https://doi.org/10.1371/journal.pone.0153715

19. Wright, M. O. D., Crawford, E., & Del Castillo, D. (2019). Childhood emotional maltreatment and later psychological distress among college students: The mediating role of maladaptive schemas. *Child Abuse & Neglect, 92*, 56–65. https://doi.org/10.1016/j.chiabu.2019.03.008

20. Finkelhor, D., Shattuck, A., Turner, H. A., & Hamby, S. L. (2014). The lifetime prevalence of child sexual abuse and sexual assault assessed in late adolescence. *Journal of Adolescent Health, 55*(3), 329–333. https://doi.org/10.1016/j.jadohealth.2013.12.026

21. Finkelhor, D., Turner, H., & Colburn, D. (2024). The prevalence of child sexual abuse with online sexual abuse added. *Child Abuse & Neglect, 149*, 106634. https://doi.org/10.1016/j.chiabu.2024.106634

22. Gewirtz-Meydan, A., & Finkelhor, D. (2020). Sexual abuse and assault in a large national sample of children and adolescents. *Child Maltreatment, 25*(2), 203–214. https://doi.org/10.1177/1077559519873975

23. Finkelhor, D., & Shattuck, A. (2012). *Characteristics of crimes against juveniles.* Durham, NH: Crimes Against Children Research Center. http://www.unh.edu/ccrc/pdf/CV26_Revised%20Characteristics%20of%20Crimes%20against%20Juveniles_5-2-12.pdf

24. American Academy of Child & Adolescent Psychiatry. (2023). *Facts for families: Child sexual abuse.* https://www.aacap.org/AACAP/Families_and_Youth/Facts_for_Families/FFF-Guide/Child-Sexual-Abuse-009.aspx

25. Child Welfare Information Gateway (2019). *Long-term consequences of child abuse and neglect.* U.S: Department of Health and Human Services, Children's Bureau. https://www.childwelfare.gov/pubPDFs/long_term_consequences.pdf

26. Mendelson, T., & Letourneau, E. J. (2015). Parent-focused prevention of child sexual abuse. *Prevention Science, 16*(6), 844–852. https://doi.org/10.1007/s11121-015-0553-z

27. Rudolph, J., & Zimmer-Gembeck, M. J. (2018). Reviewing the focus: A summary and critique of child-focused sexual abuse prevention. *Trauma, Violence & Abuse, 19*(5), 543–554. https://doi.org/10.1177/1524838016675478

28. Trew, S., Russell, D. H., Higgins, D. J., & Walsh, K. (2021). *Effective delivery methods and teaching strategies for child sexual abuse prevention: A rapid evidence check.* Institute of Child Protection Studies, Australian Catholic University. https://doi.org/10.26199/rdbq-xm46

29. Child Welfare Information Gateway (2013). *Acts of omission: An overview of child neglect.* U.S: Department of Health and Human Services, Children's Bureau. https://ocfcpacourts.us/wp-content/uploads/2020/06/Acts_of_Omission_000978.pdf

30. Dubowitz, H. (2013). Neglect in children. In R. E. Tremblay, M. Boivin, & R. DeV. Peters (Eds.), *Encyclopedia on early childhood development* (pp. 1–5). https://www.child-encyclopedia.com/pdf/expert/maltreatment-child/according-experts/child-neglect-overview

31. National Research Council (2014). *New directions in child abuse and neglect research.* National Academies Press. https://doi.org/10.17226/18331

32. Feeding America. (2023). *Map the meal gap: Food insecurity in the United States.* https://www.feedingamerica.org/research/map-the-meal-gap

33. U.S. Census Bureau. (2023). *Income and poverty in the United States: 2022.* https://www.census.gov/library/publications/2023/demo/p60-279.html

34. Heard-Garris, N., Boyd, R., Kan, K., Perez-Cardona, L., Heard, N. J., & Johnson, T. J. (2021). Structuring Poverty: How Racism Shapes Child Poverty and Child and Adolescent Health. *Academic Pediatrics, 21*(8S), S108–S116. https://doi.org/10.1016/j.acap.2021.05.026

35. Bailey, Z. D., Feldman, J. M., & Bassett, M. T. (2021). How structural racism works—Racist policies as a root cause of U.S. racial health inequities. *New England Journal of Medicine, 384*(8), 768–773. https://doi.org/10.1056/NEJMms2025396

36. Knifton, L., & Inglis, G. (2020). Poverty and mental health: policy, practice and research implications. *BJPsych Bulletin, 44*(5), 193–196. https://doi.org/10.1192/bjb.2020.78

37. Cronholm, P. F., Forke, C. M., Wade, R., Bair-Merritt, M. H., Davis, M., Harkins-Schwarz, M., ... Fein, J. A. (2015). Adverse childhood experiences: Expanding the concept of adversity. *American Journal of Preventive Medicine, 49*(3), 354–361. https://doi.org/10.1016/j.amepre.2015.02.001

38. Lacey, R. E., Minnis, H., & Pillas, D. (2020). Practitioner review: Twenty years of research with adverse childhood experience scores – Advantages, disadvantages and applications to practice. *Journal of Child Psychology and Psychiatry, 61*(2), 116–130. https://doi.org/10.1111/jcpp.13135

39. National Scientific Council on the Developing Child. (2012). *The science of neglect: The persistent absence of responsive care disrupts the developing brain* (Working Paper No. 12). Harvard University, Center on the Developing Child. https://developingchild.harvard.edu/resources/the-science-of-neglect/

40. Stoltenborgh, M., Bakermans-Kranenburg, M. J., & van IJzendoorn, M. H. (2013). The neglect of child neglect: A meta-analytic review of the prevalence of neglect. *Social Psychiatry and Psychiatric Epidemiology*, *48*(3), 345–355. https://doi.org/10.1007/s00127-012-0549-y

41. McLaughlin, K. A., Sheridan, M. A., & Lambert, H. K. (2014). Childhood adversity and neural development: Deprivation and threat as distinct dimensions of early experience. *Neuroscience & Biobehavioral Reviews*, *47*, 578–591. https://doi.org/10.1016/j.neubiorev.2014.10.012

42. Wright, M. O. D., Crawford, E., & Del Castillo, D. (2009). Childhood emotional maltreatment and later psychological distress among college students: The mediating role of maladaptive schemas. *Child Abuse & Neglect*, *33*(1), 59–68. https://doi.org/10.1016/j.chiabu.2008.12.007

43. Narayan, A. J., Rivera, L. M., Bernstein, R. E., Harris, W. W., & Lieberman, A. F. (2018). Positive childhood experiences predict less psychopathology and stress in pregnant women with childhood adversity: A pilot study of the benevolent childhood experiences (BCEs) scale. *Child Abuse & Neglect*, *78*, 19–30. https://doi.org/10.1016/j.chiabu.2017.09.022

44. Mennen, F. E., Trickett, P. K., Kim, K., & Sang, J. (2010). Child neglect: Definition and identification of youth's experiences in official reports of maltreatment. *Child Abuse & Neglect*, *34*(9), 647–658. https://doi.org/10.1016/j.chiabu.2010.02.007

45. American Psychiatric Association (2022). *Diagnostic and statistical manual of mental disorders* (5th ed., text rev.).). NIMH. https://doi.org/10.1176/appi.books.9780890425787

46. National Institute of Mental Health. (2022). *Mental illness.* https://www.nimh.nih.gov/health/statistics/mental-illness

47. National Collaborating Centre for Mental Health (Great Britain), National Institute for Health and Clinical Excellence (Great Britain), British Psychological Society, & Royal College of Psychiatrists (2011). *Common mental health disorders: Identification and pathways to care.* British Psychological Society.

48. Eylem, O., de Wit, L., van Straten, A., Steubl, L., Melissourgaki, Z., Danışman, G. T., ... Cuijpers, P. (2020). Stigma for common mental disorders in racial minorities and majorities: A systematic review and meta-analysis. *BMC Public Health*, *20*(1), 879. https://doi.org/10.1186/s12889-020-08964-0

49. Barker, E. (2022, January 12). *How to support a child when a parent has a mental illness.* Boston Children's El Hospital https://answers.childrenshospital.org/parental-mental-illness/

50. National Coalition Against Domestic Violence. (n.d.). *Domestic violence statistics.* https://ncadv.org/STATISTICS

51. Black, M. C., Basile, K. C., Breiding, M. J., Smith, S. G., Walters, M. L., Merrick, M. T., ... & Stevens, M. R. (2011). *The National Intimate Partner and Sexual Violence Survey: 2010 summary report.* Centers for Disease Control and Prevention. https://www.cdc.gov/violenceprevention/pdf/nisvs_report2010-a.pdf

52. Hamby, S., Finkelhor, D., Turner, H., & Ormrod, R. (2010). *Children's exposure to intimate partner violence and other family violence.* Juvenile Justice Bulletin, U.S: Department of Justice. https://www.ojp.gov/pdffiles1/ojjdp/232272.pdf

53. Office on Women's Health (n.d.). *Effects of domestic violence on children.* U.S. Department of Health & Human Services. https://www.womenshealth.gov/relationships-and-safety/domestic-violence/effects-domestic-violence-children

54. Barnardo's. (n.d.). *Effects of domestic abuse on children.* https://www.barnardos.org.uk/get-support/support-for-parents-and-carers/child-abuse-and-harm/children-affected-domestic-abuse-violence

55. Hurley, K. (2020). *The divorce rate is at a 50-year low.* Time Magazine. https://time.com/5434949/divorce-rate-children-marriage/

56. Petrelli, T. (2022). *Divorce statistics for 2022.* Petrelli Law. https://www.petrellilaw.com/divorce-statistics-for-2022/

57. Wolfinger, N. H. (2005). *Understanding the divorce cycle: The children of divorce in their own marriages.* Cambridge University Press.

58. Amato, P. R., & Keith, B. (1991). Parental divorce and the well-being of children: A meta-analysis. *Psychological Bulletin*, *110*(1), 26–46. https://doi.org/10.1037/0033-2909.110.1.26

59. Radhakrishna, A., Bou-Saada, I. E., Hunter, W. M., et al. (2001). Are father surrogates a risk factor for child maltreatment? *Child Maltreatment, 6*(4), 281–289.

60. Carson, E. A. (2014). *Prisoners in 2013*. Bureau of Justice Statistics. https://bjs.ojp.gov/content/pub/pdf/p13.pdf

61. Glaze, L. E., & Maruschak, L. M. (2010). *Parents in prison and their minor children*. Bureau of Justice Statistics. https://bjs.ojp.gov/content/pub/pdf/pptmc.pdf

62. Sykes, B. L., & Pettit, B. (2014). Mass incarceration, family complexity, and the reproduction of childhood disadvantage. *The Annals of the American Academy of Political and Social Science, 654*(1), 127–149. https://doi.org/10.1177/0002716214526345

63. Turney, K. (2014). Stress proliferation across generations? Examining the relationship between parental incarceration and childhood health. *Journal of Health and Social Behavior, 55*(3), 302–319. https://doi.org/10.1177/0022146514544173

64. Turney, K., & Haskins, A. R. (2014). Falling behind? Children's early grade retention after paternal incarceration. *Sociology of Education, 87*(4), 241–258. https://doi.org/10.1177/0038040714547086

65. Substance Abuse and Mental Health Services Administration. (2017). *Children living with parents who have a substance use disorder*. https://www.samhsa.gov/data/sites/default/files/report_3223/ShortReport-3223.html

66. Barnard, M., & McKeganey, N. (2004). The impact of parental problem drug use on children: What is the problem and what can be done to help? *Addiction, 99*(5), 552–559. https://doi.org/10.1111/j.1360-0443.2003.00664.x

67. Lander, L., Howsare, J., & Byrne, M. (2013). The impact of substance use disorders on families and children: From theory to practice. *Social Work in Public Health, 28*(3–4), 194–205. https://doi.org/10.1080/19371918.2013.759005

68. Office of the Assistant Secretary for Planning and Evaluation. (2021). *National and state estimates of children living with parents using substances*. https://aspe.hhs.gov/reports/children-living-parents-using-substances

69. American Addiction Centers. (2023). *Children of addicted parents guide: The impact of substance use disorders on families and children*. https://americanaddictioncenters.org/rehab-guide/children-of-addicted-parents

70. National Society for the Prevention of Cruelty to Children. (2021). *Parental substance misuse*. https://learning.nspcc.org.uk/children-and-families-at-risk/parental-substance-misuse

71. Raypole, C. (2022, July 28). *What to tell children about a parent's addiction*. Verywell Mind. https://www.verywellmind.com/what-to-tell-children-about-a-parents-addiction-66633

Preventing ACEs

The Forced Displacement of Abused Children

Forced displacement, or the removal of children from abusive homes, is one of the most contentious interventions in child welfare. Each year, child protective service (CPS) agencies in the United States investigate over 4 million allegations of abuse or neglect.[1] As a result, approximately 200,000 children are removed from their homes and placed into foster care (i.e., such as placement with a relative or a nonrelative caregiver who is not a biological parent). The primary goal of this intervention is to protect children by reducing their exposure to harmful environments. However, the effects of such removal are complex, nuanced, and understudied.

The benefits of removal primarily center on the immediate physical and emotional safety of the child. Exposure to chronic abuse is associated with severe and lasting consequences, including developmental delays, emotional dysregulation, and higher risks of psychiatric disorders.[2] Removal halts the cycle of trauma and can provide a stable and nurturing environment if high-quality foster care is available. In cases of severe physical or sexual abuse, removal is often the only viable path to ensure survival and recovery. Evidence suggests that child welfare systems have improved by using standardized assessments, removing fewer children, and implementing community-based methods for addressing child abuse. As a result, children spend less time in the foster care system and are more likely to be unified with their families.[3]

However, the costs of removal are multifaceted. Children removed from their homes often experience attachment disruptions, identity confusion, and multiple placements, which can exacerbate existing trauma.[4] Displaced children often face lower educational attainment, higher incarceration rates, and increased reliance on social services.[5,6] As a result, many scholars now advocate for preventative, in-home support interventions such as parenting programs, trauma-informed therapy, and economic assistance before resorting to removal.[7]

References

1. U.S. Department of Health and Human Services. (2016). *Child maltreatment 2016.* Administration for Children and Families, Children's Bureau. https://www.acf.hhs.gov/cb/report/child-maltreatment-2016

2. Committee on Child Maltreatment Research, Policy, and Practice for the Next Decade: Phase II, Board on Children, Youth, and Families, Committee on Law and Justice, Institute of Medicine, & National Research Council (2014). Chapter 5 The Child Welfare System. In A. C. Petersen, J. Joseph, & M. Feit (Eds.), *New directions in child abuse and neglect research* (pp. 175–244). National Academies Press. https://doi.org/10.17226/18331

3. Taylor, E. (2013). Trends in child welfare reform. *The Future of Children, 23*(2), 59–76. https://doi.org/10.1353/foc.2013.0013

4. Dozier, M., Bick, J., & Bernard, K. (2006). Enhancing the early caregiving environment to promote children's mental health: The early intervention program. *Journal of Child Psychology and Psychiatry, 47*(3–4), 349–361. https://doi.org/10.1111/j.1469-7610.2006.01649.x

5. Gypen, L., Vanderfaeillie, J., De Maeyer, S., Belenger, L., & Van Holen, F. (2017). Outcomes of children who grew up in foster care: Systematic-review. *Children and Youth Services Review, 76*, 74–83. https://doi.org/10.1016/j.childyouth.2017.02.035

6. Peterson, C., Florence, C., & Klevens, J. (2018). The economic burden of child maltreatment in the United States, 2015. *Child Abuse & Neglect, 86*, 178–183. https://doi.org/10.1016/j.chiabu.2018.09.018

7. Doyle, J. J., & Aizer, A. (2018). Economics of child protection: Maltreatment, foster care, and intimate partner violence. *Annual Review of Economics, 10*, 87–108. https://doi.org/10.1146/annurev-economics-080217-053237

Systemic Racism and Classism as Contributors to ACEs

Systemic racism and classism are deeply entrenched societal structures that significantly contribute to the prevalence and severity of ACEs. These structural inequalities shape environments that increase exposure to chronic stressors, disrupt familial stability, and limit access to critical resources, exacerbating the impact of ACEs and perpetuating intergenerational cycles of adversity.[1]

Systemic Racism and ACEs

Systemic racism manifests through policies and practices that uphold inequities in housing, education, employment, and healthcare. Historically, discriminatory practices like redlining have confined many Black and Brown families to underresourced neighborhoods marked by poverty, violence, and instability.[2] These environments increase the likelihood of children experiencing ACEs, including neglect and community violence. In underfunded schools serving marginalized communities, disparities in resources lead to overcrowded classrooms and limited access to mental health services, compounding stress for children and families.[3] In the healthcare system, families of color often face barriers to accessing preventive care and trauma-informed mental health services, leaving children more vulnerable to the long-term consequences of ACEs.[1,3]

Classism and ACEs

Classism, which privileges individuals with wealth and marginalizes those in poverty, further compounds the prevalence of ACEs. Economic insecurity imposes chronic stress on caregivers, often leading to harsh or inconsistent parenting, increasing the risk of abuse or neglect.[4] Families living in poverty are more likely to reside in substandard housing, be exposed to environmental hazards and violence, and face frequent relocations, all of which undermine children's sense of safety and stability.

Intersection of Systemic Racism and Classism

The intersection of systemic racism and classism creates compounded vulnerabilities, particularly for children from marginalized racial and socioeconomic backgrounds. Black, Indigenous, and other people of color (BIPOC) are disproportionately represented among families experiencing poverty, due to both historical injustices and current systemic inequities.[5] This dual marginalization increases exposure to multiple ACEs, including parental incarceration, exposure to community violence, and family separation or involvement in the child welfare system.[6]

Educational Disparities and ACEs

Educational disparities deepen the impact of ACEs. Students who have experienced multiple adversities are more likely to struggle academically and exhibit emotional and behavioral challenges, such as anxiety, aggression, or difficulty concentrating. These difficulties often result in lower academic achievement and reduced life opportunities, reinforcing the cycle of trauma and disadvantage.[3,4]

Addressing Structural Inequities

To mitigate ACEs, efforts must go beyond individual treatment and address the broader structural inequities that perpetuate them. Policy recommendations include expanding affordable housing, investing in desegregated and equitably funded schools, enforcing anti-discrimination hiring practices, and ensuring universal access to affordable healthcare and mental health services.[1,7] Addressing these inequities on a system level can break cycles of abuse and provide structural support for children to thrive.

References

1. Salud America. (2022). *FAQ: Racism is a public health crisis.* https://salud-america.org/wp-content/uploads/2022/02/FAQ-Racism-is-a-Public-Health-Crisis-2022.pdf

2. Bailey, Z. D., Feldman, J. M., & Bassett, M. T. (2021). How structural racism works—racist policies as a root cause of U.S. racial health inequities. *New England Journal of Medicine, 384*(8), 768–773. https://doi.org/10.1056/NEJMms2025396

3. Financial Times. (2023). *Unequal school funding hobbles the American dream.* https://www.ft.com/content/28e923e2-d934-4aa0-8cbe-2d6f4b2f4014

4. Murphey, D., & Sacks, V. (2019). The prevalence of adverse childhood experiences, nationally and by state. *American Educator, Summer 2019.* https://www.aft.org/ae/summer2019/murphey_sacks

5. Connell, C. M., Vanderploeg, J. J., Katz, K. H., Caron, C., Saunders, L., & Tebes, J. K. (2019). *The intersectionality of adverse childhood experiences, race/ethnicity, and income: Implications for policy.* ResearchGate.

6. Cronholm, P. F., Forke, C. M., Wade, R., Bair-Merritt, M. H., Davis, M., Harkins-Schwarz, M., ... Fein, J. A. (2015). Adverse childhood experiences: Expanding the concept of adversity. *American Journal of Preventive Medicine, 49*(3), 354–361.

7. The Guardian. (2024). *Structural racism leading to stark health inequalities in London.* https://www.theguardian.com/world/2024/oct/01/structural-racism-leading-to-stark-health-inequalities-in-london-report-shows

ACEs and the Brain: The Basics

Scientists have long understood the impact of trauma on behavior and are beginning to understand the influence of ACEs on a chemical level in the brain. Individuals with multiple ACEs face an elevated risk of developing mental health and physical conditions. While various factors contribute to this heightened risk, one factor could be the physical impact of stressful experiences on the brain.

When consistently exposed to fear or stress, their brain may adapt to survive this challenging environment. This adaptation might lead to the impaired development of brain regions responsible for logical thinking, like the prefrontal cortex (PFC), and memory, such as the hippocampus. Conversely, brain regions involved in emotional responses, like the amygdala, become more active, increasing vigilance to potential threats. These changes can result in difficulties in regulating emotions, making decisions, and managing stress. These challenges can manifest in depression, anxiety, substance abuse, and other mental illnesses.

Childhood trauma has also been linked to poorer physical health. ACEs impact the stress response systems. When these systems malfunction, it contributes to free radicals and antioxidants in the brain, which lowers the immune system. As a result, children and adults with a history of childhood trauma tend to have a higher prevalence of acute and chronic physical ailments. Additionally, they may engage in risky behaviors that exacerbate these conditions, such as smoking, substance abuse, and unhealthy diet and exercise habits that can contribute to obesity. In turn, there is an increased susceptibility to physical diseases such as cancer, diabetes, and heart disease.

The extent to which these events affect a person depends on their genetics and environment. For instance, someone may experience multiple ACEs but possess genetic resilience to stress. Furthermore, these changes in the brain are not necessarily permanent. The brain retains its capacity to adapt and change throughout childhood and adulthood, allowing areas that may have been affected by specific events to strengthen over time.

Engaging in activities like exercise, socializing, and mindfulness exercises has been shown to enhance the functioning of frontal brain areas, including the PFC. Additionally, optimal PFC functioning can be promoted through self-care practices such as getting sufficient sleep and avoiding excessive drug and alcohol use.

Recovery From ACEs

ACEs and Positive Childhood Experiences

Many things contribute to resilience and protect from the worst outcomes of ACEs. This can include critical thinking skills, social competency, spirituality, and other supportive, healthy adults. We may not be able to control our innate abilities, but there are some things we can seek out. For example, science suggests that supportive and nurturing relationships with caring adults and friends can offset the impact of ACEs.[1] These adults provide the emotional stability, guidance, and validation that are crucial for resilience, helping to buffer the trauma and create a foundation for healing and growth.

Individuals with three to seven positive childhood experiences (PCEs) tend to have fewer poor mental health days and depression.[1] According to Bethell and colleagues, the seven PCEs include:

❑ Felt able to talk to family about feelings
❑ Felt their family stood by them during difficult times
❑ Enjoyed participating in community traditions
❑ Felt a sense of belonging in high school (not including those who did not attend school or were home-schooled)

❑   Felt supported by friends
❑   Had at least two nonparent adults who took genuine interest in them
❑   Felt safe and protected by an adult in their home

While society seeks solutions to reduce ACEs, it would also be helpful to increase PCEs. Identifying school, community, and friendship connections and other caring adults can help build resilience for ACEs survivors. Assessing for ACEs only is a deficit approach, and providers should evaluate for individual strengths and assets. These assets can inform specialized interventions and reduce the likelihood of ACEs' negative mental, social, and physical health consequences.

Reference

1. Bethell, C. D., Jones, J., Gombojav, N., Linkenbach, J., & Sege, R. (2019). Positive childhood experiences and adult mental and relational health in a statewide sample: Associations across adverse childhood experiences levels. *JAMA Pediatrics*, *173*(11), e193007. https://doi.org/10.1001/jamapediatrics.2019.3007

Healthy Coping Strategies

- *Talk to Someone Safe:* Think of someone in your life who you respect, trust, and who makes you feel good about yourself. This could be a friend, relative, teacher, mentor, coach, or anyone who looks out for you in a healthy way. Talk to these trusted adults about your problems, fears, and needs. A caring confidant can help you deal with your issues and build resilience.

- *Connect with Healthy Friends and Family:* One of the greatest tools of abuse is isolation. Isolation leaves you alone to question yourself and perhaps your sanity. It blocks you from outside perspectives that may help you deal with your abuse. It is tempting to hide abuse. You may feel embarrassed or frightened, but the abuser is the one who should have these feelings. Please don't turn away from friends or supportive family; lean on them in times of crisis.

- *Keep a Journal of Your Feelings and Events:* I am a strong advocate for journaling. Journaling gave me a record of key points in my life that served as the foundation for this book. Journals can be written in notebooks, diaries, or online (e.g., email, blog). You could use a video diary or write poetry, raps, or songs if you are more artistic. Sharing your story, even privately, is a great way to work through your problems.

- *Participate in Healthy Activities:* Finding activities that you enjoy can distract you and make you feel good. Think about things that you like to do. Hobbies such as reading, dancing, gaming, or shopping may be of interest. Social activities might include hanging out with friends, family, or pets. There are also sensory experiences that you may find pleasurable, such as warm baths, relaxing music, or knitting/crocheting. Exercise and movement can also be pleasurable. Spend more time doing things that bring you joy.

- *Create a Safety Plan:* A safety plan is essential if you live with an abusive parent, caregiver, or partner. A safety plan is a list of steps to increase your security in the event of future abuse. First, you need to get to a safe place. It is vital to get away from the violence and avoid further danger. Think about where you could go and keep a list of those locations. If possible, find a secure room away from your abuser or leave and go to a safer location (e.g., neighbor, family, friends, teen shelter, library, park). Always let a trusted person know where you are. Keep money on hand to use a pay phone or take a bus. Keep a list of people you can call for help, such as the trusted person identified above, a concerned neighbor, support hotlines, or the authorities.

- *Read Self-help Books:* Psychology self-help books can offer several benefits for individuals seeking personal growth, self-improvement, and a better understanding of their mental and emotional well-being. It's important to note that while psychology self-help books can be beneficial, they are not a substitute for professional mental health treatment when needed. Additionally, the effectiveness of self-help books can vary from person to person, so it's essential to find resources that resonate with your individual needs and preferences.

- *Remember That It's Not Your Fault:* No matter what anyone says, especially your abuser, abuse is never your fault. You are not even partially to blame. You do not deserve it. Abusers may try to convince you that their actions are because of something you did or didn't do. Even if you misbehave as a child, it's up to your parents/caregivers to discipline you appropriately. Abusers are great at manipulating others into thinking that they are the cause of all of their problems. You are not in charge of other people's behavior. Verbal abuse and physical assaults are never appropriate, no matter what your family, culture, or religion might say. You cannot make a person abusive or violent. It is their choice and their behavior that needs to change. Abuse is dangerous and against the law. It should be reported if doing so will keep others safe.

Help-Seeking Stigma

The stigma around mental health can discourage individuals from seeking the care they need, leading to delayed or avoided treatment, which can cause a deterioration of their mental health. Mental health professionals create a safe and nonjudgmental space where clients can feel heard and understood as they process their experiences. Therapy offers increased self-awareness, enhanced problem-solving, and coping skills.

There is absolutely no shame in seeking therapy. Recognizing the need for professional support and taking steps to prioritize your mental health is a courageous and empowering decision. In fact, seeking therapy reflects a commitment to your well-being and personal growth. Just as we consult healthcare professionals for physical ailments, seeking therapy is a proactive and constructive way to address mental and emotional challenges. It demonstrates strength, self-awareness, and a willingness to invest in your own mental health. However, it is important especially when dealing with trauma to seek a qualified mental health provider.

What Is a Qualified Mental Health Professional?

I was at a party once where the host excitedly introduced me to "another clinical psychologist." I was immediately eager to make a new professional connection and began asking the usual questions. Where do you work? Where did you train? Her response to those two basic questions told me instantly that she wasn't a psychologist. In California and most other states, a psychologist has a doctorate, thousands of hours of supervised professional experience, and has passed a series of professional and ethics exams. My questions had inadvertently outed her. She began to backpedal and clarify that she had a master's in applied psychology and had worked as a coach for business executives. To the untrained eye, her advanced degree in a field that sounded clinical gave her perceived credibility as a clinical psychologist when she wasn't.

Unfortunately, this is a common occurrence. While there are a range of useful helping professionals, it is important to practice within the scope of our professional limits. Screening, assessment, and treatment for psychological disorders and trauma should be done under the care of a qualified licensed mental health professional.

Trained mental health professionals undergo rigorous education, often obtaining advanced degrees in clinical fields such as clinical psychology, counseling, social work, or psychiatry. This academic foundation equips them with a comprehensive understanding of the complexities of human behavior, mental health theories, and evidence-based therapeutic techniques.

Clinical training further refines their skills, allowing mental health professionals to apply theoretical knowledge in practical settings. This hands-on experience is invaluable, fostering the development of therapeutic skills, interpersonal competence, and the ability to navigate diverse client needs.

Licensure is a crucial aspect that distinguishes mental health professionals from others who may lack the necessary qualifications. Obtaining a license involves meeting specific educational and clinical requirements, passing rigorous examinations, and adhering to ethical standards. This official endorsement ensures that practitioners are held to a recognized standard of competence and ethical conduct, providing an additional layer of assurance for those seeking mental health support. Finding a therapist, the right therapist, can be tricky. Here are some steps to help you:

- *Assess Your Needs:* Start by identifying your specific needs and goals for therapy. Consider the issues you want to address, whether you prefer individual or group therapy, and any particular preferences like gender or culture.
- *Consult Your Insurance:* If you have health insurance, check your policy to understand your mental health coverage. Make a note of any in-network therapists to help with cost considerations.
- *Ask for Recommendations:* Seek recommendations from trusted sources, such as friends, family members, or healthcare professionals. They may know of therapists with a good reputation.
- *Use Online Resources:* Explore online directories and resources dedicated to finding therapists (see Resources).
- *Contact Your Primary Care Physician:* Your primary care doctor can provide referrals to mental health specialists and help coordinate your care. Sometimes, they have therapists on site.
- *Research Therapists:* Look into therapists' backgrounds, qualifications, areas of expertise, and reviews if available. Ensure they are licensed and have relevant experience in treating your specific concerns.

- *Consider Accessibility:* Evaluate the location, hours of availability, and whether the therapist offers in-person or virtual sessions to ensure it aligns with your needs and schedule.
- *Interview Potential Therapists:* Contact therapists to ask questions about their approach to therapy, treatment methods, fees, and availability. It is best not to provide too many details of your experiences at this stage to increase your odds of getting a callback. Also, if they are unavailable, ask for additional referrals.
- *Trust Your Instincts:* Trust your gut feeling when choosing a therapist. A solid therapeutic alliance and a sense of comfort and trust with your therapist are crucial for effective therapy. Move on if you don't mesh, but communicate your intentions before you do so.
- *Schedule an Initial Session:* Arrange an initial appointment or consultation with the therapist to assess whether you feel comfortable and whether their approach aligns with your needs.
- *Assess the Therapeutic Relationship:* During the first few sessions, evaluate your rapport with the therapist. Openly communicate your expectations and goals for therapy.
- *Regularly Review Progress:* Continually assess your progress and the effectiveness of therapy. If you feel that therapy is not meeting your needs, consider discussing this with your therapist or seeking a second opinion.

Finding the right therapist may take time, but it's crucial to achieving your mental health goals. Don't hesitate to seek support and guidance from multiple sources during this process.

Treatment for ACEs

A trained mental health professional will conduct a clinical assessment to determine the most appropriate therapeutic interventions. It's important to note that the treatment approach may vary depending on the individual's specific needs and the severity of their ACEs. Mental health professionals can employ various therapeutic approaches to help individuals who have had ACEs. The goal of treatment is to address ACEs' emotional and psychological impact and support individuals in their healing process. Cognitive behavioral therapy (CBT) seems to be the most effective treatment modality for adults recovering from ACEs.[1,2] Other therapies to consider include trauma-informed therapies, emotion-focused therapy, and mindfulness-based therapy; however, the results are inconclusive.[1,2]

Individual, family, or group counseling sessions provide a safe space for individuals to explore their experiences, express their feelings, and develop a deeper understanding of how ACEs have affected their lives. In some cases, a multidisciplinary approach involving therapists, psychiatrists, social workers, and other professionals may be necessary to address various aspects of ACE-related issues.

Therapy may be a long-term process, as healing from ACEs can take time, patience, and require ongoing support. Case complexity, difficulty establishing trust, and generation patterns can make the process more challenging. It's essential to maintain open communication with your therapist, set realistic expectations, and commit to the therapeutic process to achieve the best possible outcomes.

References

1. Korotana, L. M., Dobson, K. S., Pusch, D., & Josephson, T. (2016). A review of primary care interventions to improve health outcomes in adult survivors of adverse childhood experiences. *Clinical Psychology Review, 46,* 59–90. https://doi.org/10.1016/j.cpr.2016.04.007
2. Lorenc, T., Lester, S., Sutcliffe, K., Stansfield, C., Thomas, J., & Harden, A. (2020). Interventions to support people exposed to adverse childhood experiences: Systematic review of systematic reviews. *BMC Public Health, 20,* 657. https://doi.org/10.1186/s12889-020-08789-0

Post-traumatic Growth

Post-traumatic growth (PTG) is a theory developed in the mid-1990s that explains the positive changes that can occur in individuals after facing psychological struggles following adversity.[1] One research study suggests that almost half of trauma survivors experience growth after a traumatic experience.[2] According to PTG theory, people who endure challenges often experience personal growth across five domains.

1. **Appreciation of Life:**
   - *Before:* Taking life for granted, not fully appreciating everyday moments.
   - *After PTG:* Developing a deep gratitude for life, finding joy in small things, and cherishing the present moment.

2. **Relationships with Others:**
   - *Before:* Struggling with trust, difficulty forming meaningful connections.
   - *After PTG:* Cultivating stronger, more authentic relationships, with an increased ability to empathize and connect emotionally.

3. **New Possibilities in Life:**
   - *Before:* Feeling stuck or limited by circumstances.
   - *After PTG:* Recognizing opportunities for growth and change, being open to new experiences and challenges.

4. **Personal Strength:**
   - *Before:* Perceiving oneself as weak or powerless.
   - *After PTG:* Discovering inner resilience, a sense of personal strength, and the ability to overcome adversity.

5. **Spiritual Change:**
   - *Before:* Little or no engagement with spirituality or a sense of purpose.
   - *After PTG:* Finding a deeper meaning in life, experiencing spiritual growth, and developing a stronger sense of purpose or connection to something greater than oneself.

Recognizing that challenging experiences can act as a catalyst for positive growth might inspire hope for those navigating recovery. Nonetheless, it is crucial not to downplay the impact of your trauma. Taking the necessary time to genuinely process it, rather than hastily seeking a superficial sense of optimism, is important. Adversity can lead to positive changes that contribute to a richer and more fulfilling life.

References

1. Tedeschi, R. G., Shakespeare-Finch, J., Taku, K., & Calhoun, L. G. (2018). *Posttraumatic growth: Theory, research, and applications.* Routledge.
2. Wu, X., Kaminga, A. C., Dai, W., Deng, J., Wang, Z., Pan, X., & Liu, A. (2019). The prevalence of moderate-to-high posttraumatic growth: A systematic review and meta-analysis. *Journal of Affective Disorders, 243,* 408–415. https://doi.org/10.1016/j.jad.2018.09.023

Acknowledgements

TO MY DAUGHTERS, who inspired me to pursue a better life for my children long before they were born. I have tried to undo my legacy to set the stage for a more promising future for you and yours. *I love you to pieces.*

To my dearest Damien, my rock and partner in life. You've been a steadfast ally and unwavering defender, standing by my side through thick and thin. Your unwavering support has been my shield and your selflessness, truly admirable. Thank you for being not just a buffer but a willing sacrificial lamb, always there when I needed you the most.

With heartfelt thanks to Dev, my cherished sister and best friend. You walked beside me through the darkest times of our childhood and I wouldn't have made it without you. I hate knowing the senseless pain you suffered— you didn't deserve it either. I have always felt like I understood you and had a great empathy for you. I am so proud that you've made your own path in your own time. Our bond has remained resilient and unbreakable through it all. *Me and you, us never part.*

To my beloved siblings, I aspire for this book to offer you a deeper insight into my life and perspective. Even more importantly, I hope it serves as a mirror for you to reflect upon yourself and continue to grow. Let us collectively commit to no longer allowing external influences to shape the essence of our relationships.

Thank you to my uncles, Brian and Joey. Uncle Brian, I want to express my profound gratitude to you for undertaking one of the most challenging tasks within a family—speaking the unvarnished truth. Your courage and honesty paved the way for our escape, for my escape. Moreover, your unwavering support and encouragement empowered me to share my story with the world, with the hope that it might inspire others to realize that their beginnings need not define their destinies. Through your support, I have discovered my own bravery. Uncle Joe, you gave me my very first job as a babysitter. You and Aunt Heidi's house was another safe haven in my life and your generosity provided much needed financial support. From the day I was admitted into grad school, and you affectionately started calling me "doc," I felt a sense of encouragement and motivation that boosted my confidence.

(dis)Honor Thy Mother: Daughterhood, Dysfunction and Deliverance, First Edition. Bridgette Peteet.
© 2026 John Wiley & Sons, Inc. Published 2026 by John Wiley & Sons, Inc.

To the rest of my family. I love you. I recognize that reading this book may have been a challenging experience. However, my ultimate hope is that you can see beyond any discomfort and grasp the larger purpose—the imperative need to spare others from enduring abuse in silence and to offer them a chance to begin to heal.

I am forever grateful for my girlfriends, in-laws, mentors, coworkers, and sorority sisters. There are too many to name and I'd certainly fail in trying to list them all. You are a cadre of compassionate individuals, many of whom are also in helping professions. You all provided me with a lot of free supplemental "therapy" sessions over the years to help me unravel a complicated past, minimize my defenses, and told me the truth when I needed to hear it. I've observed your strength and wisdom with unwavering attention, and I've borrowed more from each of you than you could ever imagine.

Thank you to the faithful members of my virtual book writer's workgroup, Drs. Stacey Williams, Clare Mehta, Emily Keener, and Shannon Audley, for your feedback, resources and encouragement over the years. Readers, you must buy all of their books too.

This memoir is also dedicated to the cherished memory of Granny. Her boundless love, unconditional nurturing, and unwavering acceptance served as the foundation of my healing. Along with Pawpaw, their timely embrace during a pivotal moment in my life allowed me to prioritize school over mere survival. They sowed the seeds of faith within me, furnishing an additional wellspring of strength. My gratitude for them could fill volumes. This book will have to do.